Cephalexin Antibiotic

THE COMPLETE CEPHALEXIN GUIDE

A Detailed Treatment for UTIs, Ear Infections, Sinusitis, and Other Bacterial Conditions with Practical Guidance on Dosage, Usage, and Potential Side Effects

JEAN LIZAH

Copyright © [2024] Jean Lizah. All rights reserved.

This publication, including its illustrations, design, and text, is protected by copyright law. No part of this book may be reproduced, stored in a retrieval system, or transmitted in any form or by any means—electronic, mechanical, photocopying, recording, or otherwise—without prior written permission from the author.

Disclaimer

This book is intended for informational purposes only and does not serve as a substitute for professional medical advice, diagnosis, or treatment. The information contained herein is based on the author's research and experience, and while every effort has been made to ensure accuracy, it may not be applicable to every individual or situation.

Readers are encouraged to seek the advice of qualified healthcare professionals for any questions or concerns regarding their health or medical conditions. This book does not prescribe or promote the use of cephalexin or any other medication. It is designed to provide valuable insights into the applications, mechanisms, and considerations associated with this antibiotic, particularly in the treatment of bacterial infections.

The content of this book should not be construed as medical advice or a recommendation for any specific treatment. Always consult a healthcare provider before starting or altering any medication regimen.

The author and publisher disclaim any liability for any direct, indirect, or consequential damages resulting from the use of this book or reliance on the information provided herein.

Table of Content

THE COMPLETE..1
CEPHALEXIN GUIDE..1
Chapter 1...15
Understanding Cephalexin...15
   1.1 What Is Cephalexin?... 18
   1.2 How It Works in the Body......................................20
   1.3 Common Uses and Approved Indications........23
CHAPTER 2..27
When Is Cephalexin Prescribed?...................................27
   2.1 Treating Bacterial Infections............................. 30
   2.2 Conditions It Covers (Respiratory, Skin, UTI, and More)..33
   2.3 Who Should and Shouldn't Use Cephalexin....37
CHAPTER 3..41
How to Take Cephalexin Safely.....................................41
   3.1 Dosage Guidelines for Adults and Children.... 45
   3.2 What to Expect During Treatment................... 48
   3.3 Importance of Completing the Course............51
CHAPTER 4..56
Potential Side Effects and Risks................................... 56
   4.1 Common Side Effects.. 60
   4.2 Recognizing Allergic Reactions........................63
   4.3 When to Contact a Doctor.................................66
CHAPTER 5..70
Drug Interactions and Precautions..............................70
   5.1 Medications That May Interact with

    Cephalexin..74
    5.2 Impact of Alcohol and Food on Effectiveness 78
    5.3 Managing Pre-Existing Conditions.................... 81
CHAPTER 6... 85
Cephalexin for Specific Infections................................ 85
    6.1 Skin Infections and Wound Care....................... 88
    6.2 Urinary Tract Infections (UTIs).........................92
    6.3 Respiratory Infections (Sinusitis, Bronchitis).95
CHAPTER 7... 100
Cephalexin vs. Other Antibiotics................................ 100
    7.1 How It Compares to Other Common Antibiotics 103
    7.2 When Cephalexin Is Preferred........................... 107
CHAPTER 8... 111
Consulting Your Healthcare Provider........................ 111
    8.1 Questions to Ask Before Taking Cephalexin.. 114
    8.2 Monitoring Progress and Follow-Up............... 118
    8.3 What to Do If Symptoms Persist...................... 121
CHAPTER 9... 125
Lifestyle Tips During Antibiotic Treatment.............. 125
    9.1 Importance of Hydration and Rest...................129
    9.2 Foods That Support Recovery........................... 132
    9.3 Managing Digestive Side Effects......................135
CHAPTER 10.. 139
Dealing with Missed or Incorrect Doses.................... 139
    10.1 What to Do If You Miss a Dose........................ 142
    10.2 Handling Overdoses Safely............................... 145
    10.3 Avoiding Antibiotic Resistance....................... 148
CHAPTER 11...152

Myths and Misconceptions About Antibiotics......... 152
    11.1 Understanding Antibiotic Resistance............ 156
    11.2 Are All Infections Treatable with Antibiotics?... 160
    11.3 Clearing Up Confusion About Side Effects...163

CHAPTER 12..168

Cephalexin in Special Populations...............................168
    12.1 Use in Children.. 171
    12.2 Use During Pregnancy and Breastfeeding....175
    12.3 Use in Elderly Patients......................................178

CHAPTER 13..183

Future of Antibiotic Treatments..................................183

INTRODUCTION

Imagine this: You wake up feeling a bit off—your throat is sore, maybe there's some swelling, and you've got a fever creeping in. You head to the doctor, and after a quick checkup, they hand you a prescription for an antibiotic: Cephalexin. At that moment, you might not give much thought to the tiny capsules you'll soon be swallowing, but those pills have a story. And understanding that story could make a big difference in how you take your medication and what you expect along the way.

Cephalexin is one of those antibiotics that many people encounter without realizing how common it is. It's prescribed for a variety of infections—anything from a persistent skin infection to a urinary tract infection (UTI) that just won't quit. If you've ever had a minor wound that got a little red and puffy or needed help kicking a sinus infection, there's a good chance Cephalexin could have been part of the solution.

But antibiotics like Cephalexin aren't just about "getting rid of the bad bugs." They come with responsibilities—completing the course, managing side effects, and knowing when to call the doctor if things don't go as planned. You might have heard about antibiotic resistance or wondered why you need to keep taking the pills even when you feel better. That's where this book comes in: to answer those questions, clear up misconceptions, and help you feel more confident using this medication.

Think of this guide as your friendly companion on the journey through treatment. Whether you're taking Cephalexin for the first time or just want to understand it better, we'll walk through everything step-by-step, making sure nothing feels overwhelming. Along the way, we'll share practical tips, real-life examples, and stories that might feel familiar—like a parent managing their child's infection or someone recovering from surgery without complications thanks to the right antibiotics.

By the end, you'll have a deeper understanding of what Cephalexin does, how to use it effectively, and how to recognize when it's doing its job (or when it's not). So, let's start this journey together. After all, knowing what's inside those little pills and how they work gives you the power to take care of yourself with confidence and ease.

Why This Book on Cephalexin?

Why write a whole book on Cephalexin, you might wonder? After all, it's just another antibiotic, right? But if you've ever had to take it—or watched a loved one go through a course of treatment—you know that taking medication isn't always as straightforward as it seems. Questions often pop up: Why do I need to finish the whole bottle if I already feel better? Is it okay to drink alcohol while on it? What happens if I miss a dose? These are the small but important things that can make a big difference in your experience with the drug.

Many of us only think about antibiotics when we're not feeling our best. Maybe it's a parent scrambling to get their child's ear infection under control, or someone battling a nagging UTI that flares up at the worst possible moment. Or perhaps you've had surgery, and your doctor handed you a prescription for Cephalexin to prevent an infection you can't even see. These are common scenarios, but the information we get from quick visits to the doctor or pharmacist can feel rushed, leaving us with more questions than answers.

This book was written to bridge that gap. We're here to go beyond the prescription label and help you truly understand what Cephalexin is, how it works, and how to make the most of it. Whether you're taking it now or want to be prepared for the next time, our goal is to demystify the medication and ease any anxiety you might feel.

We've also included stories and examples that might sound familiar. Maybe your child's antibiotic had to be hidden in applesauce to get them to take it, or you're worried about getting the timing right between doses during a busy day. These real-life challenges are part of the experience, and knowing what to expect can make things a little easier.

Most importantly, we want to empower you with knowledge. Antibiotics like Cephalexin are powerful tools, but they need to be used correctly to do their job—and to avoid problems like antibiotic resistance. With this book, you'll have the information you need to use Cephalexin confidently, avoid common pitfalls, and feel in control of your treatment.

So, whether you're reading this out of curiosity or necessity, we're glad you're here. By the time you turn the last page, you'll feel more prepared, more informed, and hopefully a little more at ease with the process. After all, taking care of yourself or someone you love is already a big responsibility—understanding your medication shouldn't be one more thing to worry about.

How to Use This Guide

You might be wondering how best to navigate this book, especially if you're here because you or someone you care about is starting a course of Cephalexin. This guide isn't meant to overwhelm you with complicated medical jargon—it's designed to make things simple, practical, and easy to understand. Think of it as a friendly conversation that walks you through everything you need to know, one step at a time. Whether you're flipping through for quick answers or want to dive deeper into specific topics, this book has been structured to suit your needs.

We know life gets busy, and when you're not feeling well, the last thing you need is a dense wall of information. That's why the sections are organized so you can jump around and find what matters to you most. If you want to get straight to how to take Cephalexin safely, there's a chapter for that. If you're curious about possible side effects or drug interactions, we've got you covered too. Maybe you just want peace of mind about what to expect for your child or elderly parent—there's something in here for you.

Each section is written with real-life scenarios in mind, the kinds of moments that might make you stop and think, "Am I doing this right?" Maybe you forgot a dose because the day got away from you—should you double up or skip it? Or maybe you're worried about mixing it with your usual vitamins or that weekend glass of wine. These are common questions, and this guide is here to give you straightforward answers.

If you prefer to read the book from start to finish, that's great too! You'll get a complete picture of Cephalexin: what it is, how it works, and how to use it wisely. But if you're in a hurry or just looking for a specific tip, feel free to jump straight to the part that's most relevant to you. Think of it like flipping through a recipe book—you don't always need the whole thing; sometimes, you just need that one perfect recipe.

Throughout the book, you'll also find tips, personal anecdotes, and insights to make things more relatable. Taking an antibiotic isn't just about swallowing pills; it's about balancing treatment with daily life. Maybe you're trying to keep track of doses in between work meetings, or perhaps you're dealing with a fussy toddler who refuses to take their medicine unless it's disguised as candy. We've included these kinds of practical moments because they're part of the experience too.

Our hope is that this guide becomes a useful companion, not just a reference book. By the end, you'll feel more comfortable and confident in managing your treatment. Whether it's your first time with Cephalexin or just one of many encounters with antibiotics, this book is here to help you make sense of it all—and hopefully, make things a little less stressful along the way.

Chapter 1

Understanding Cephalexin

You might be wondering, "What exactly is Cephalexin, and why is it so commonly prescribed?" That's a good place to start because understanding how this antibiotic works can make the whole experience feel a bit less daunting. Cephalexin is part of a group of medications called cephalosporins, which might sound complicated, but here's an easy way to think about it: Imagine it as a defender on your body's team, targeting and fighting off certain bacteria that don't belong.

Doctors prescribe Cephalexin for a variety of infections—things like skin infections, respiratory issues, or urinary tract infections (UTIs). It's especially handy when dealing with common bacterial infections that can crop up unexpectedly. Picture this: a kid with a stubborn ear infection that just won't go away or an older relative battling a UTI that's making daily life miserable. In those moments, Cephalexin steps in as a reliable solution to help people feel better.

One thing to note is that Cephalexin doesn't just attack all bacteria—it's selective. That's important because not all bacteria are bad. Our bodies have good bacteria too, like the ones in our gut that help with digestion. Cephalexin focuses on the harmful ones causing the infection, giving your immune system the boost it needs to win the fight.

You might also wonder, "How does it know where to go?" While it's not magic, the way Cephalexin works is pretty amazing. After you take a dose, the medication spreads throughout your body via your bloodstream, finding the infected area. Once there, it prevents the bacteria from building the protective walls they need to survive and multiply. Without their defenses, the bacteria become vulnerable, and your immune system can step in to finish the job.

It's easy to think of antibiotics like Cephalexin as quick fixes—and they do work quickly in many cases—but understanding that they're part of a larger process helps set realistic expectations. The first few doses might make you feel a bit better, but it's crucial to complete the full course, even if you feel fine halfway through. If you stop too early, some bacteria could survive and come back stronger, possibly causing a more severe infection.

For many people, Cephalexin feels like a lifeline during frustrating health moments. It offers a sense of relief when a lingering cough, painful UTI, or persistent skin irritation just won't improve on its own. But like any medication, it's not a one-size-fits-all solution, and using it responsibly is key to keeping it effective for the long run.

In this chapter, we'll dive deeper into the details—what Cephalexin is good for, how it compares to other antibiotics, and the importance of knowing when and how to use it. By the end, you'll have a clearer understanding of how this medication fits into your treatment plan and why it has become a trusted tool for doctors worldwide.

1.1 What Is Cephalexin?

So, what exactly is Cephalexin? In simple terms, it's an antibiotic—one of those go-to medicines doctors reach for when you have a bacterial infection that needs treatment. Think of it like a firefighter, rushing in to control a small blaze before it spreads into something more dangerous. Cephalexin belongs to a family of antibiotics called cephalosporins, which work by targeting harmful bacteria and preventing them from multiplying.

You might have encountered Cephalexin without even realizing it. Have you ever had a painful skin infection or a stubborn urinary tract infection (UTI) that wouldn't budge until you got a prescription? That's where Cephalexin comes in—helping to calm things down and clear out the bacteria causing trouble.

Cephalexin works in a straightforward way. Once you take a dose, it spreads throughout your body and zeroes in on the infection. It stops the bacteria from building protective walls, making them easy targets for your immune system. Imagine trying to build a sandcastle without any water to hold the sand together—that's what bacteria experience when Cephalexin does its job. One of the reasons Cephalexin is so widely used is that it treats a variety of infections. From sore throats caused by strep to minor skin issues like impetigo, it's a versatile option. It's often prescribed for respiratory infections, UTIs, and skin infections, especially when doctors want to avoid more aggressive antibiotics.

You might wonder, "Why not just use the same antibiotic for everything?" That's a great question. The truth is, not all antibiotics work for every kind of bacteria. Cephalexin is particularly effective against certain types, especially the ones responsible for common infections. Doctors choose it because it's reliable and generally well-tolerated, with fewer side effects compared to some stronger antibiotics.

Another reason Cephalexin is popular is that it's considered safe for most people, including children and the elderly. Of course, every medication has its limitations, and Cephalexin is no exception. It won't work against viral infections like the flu or the common cold, which can sometimes confuse people expecting an instant fix. But when used correctly, it's a powerful tool in treating bacterial infections and getting patients back on their feet.

Understanding what Cephalexin is and how it works helps you use it more effectively. Whether it's you, your child, or an older family member taking it, knowing what's going on behind the scenes makes the whole treatment process feel less intimidating. In the next sections, we'll explore more about when doctors prescribe Cephalexin, what to expect when taking it, and how to use it responsibly for the best results.

1.2 How It Works in the Body

When you take a dose of Cephalexin, you might wonder, "What exactly happens next?" The journey this antibiotic takes through your body is fascinating—and surprisingly quick. After you swallow a capsule or spoonful of liquid, Cephalexin travels through your digestive system and is absorbed into your bloodstream, ready to get to work.

Once in the bloodstream, Cephalexin acts like a skilled locksmith, targeting the bacteria causing trouble. Most bacteria have a protective wall around them, much like a brick wall shielding a fortress. Cephalexin's job is to stop the bacteria from building and repairing that wall. Without it, the bacteria become vulnerable, and your immune system steps in to finish the job. It's almost like catching burglars before they can reinforce their hideout—once exposed, they have no way to escape.

Let's imagine a common situation where Cephalexin is used, like treating a urinary tract infection (UTI). If bacteria have made their way into the bladder, it can cause burning, pain, and frequent urges to pee. Once Cephalexin reaches the infection site, it stops the bacteria from growing. As the bacteria weaken and die, symptoms like burning or pressure start to fade, and the body begins to heal.

Cephalexin works best when you take it consistently, usually every 6 to 12 hours. Think of it like watering a plant at the right times—each dose maintains the right "level" of antibiotic in your system to keep fighting off the bacteria. If you skip doses or stop taking it early, the bacteria could recover, and the infection might come back even stronger. That's why doctors always remind patients to complete the full course, even if they feel better after just a few days. Another advantage of Cephalexin is how efficiently the body handles it. Most of the medication is filtered out through the kidneys and exits the body when you urinate. This is one reason why doctors often recommend drinking extra water while on Cephalexin—staying hydrated helps your kidneys do their job and flush everything out smoothly.

It's also reassuring to know that Cephalexin doesn't just randomly attack anything in its path. It targets specific bacteria without harming the good bacteria that live peacefully in your body. Of course, every medication has some side effects, and Cephalexin can occasionally upset your stomach or cause mild diarrhea. But for most people, it's a safe and straightforward treatment option that quickly gets them back on track.

Understanding how Cephalexin works can help you use it more confidently. Knowing that each dose plays a role in clearing the infection might encourage you to stick with the full course, even when you start feeling better halfway through. It's all about timing and consistency—just like following a recipe to get the perfect dish. With Cephalexin working behind the scenes, your body has the upper hand in clearing out infections and keeping you healthy.

1.3 Common Uses and Approved Indications

You might wonder, "When exactly do doctors prescribe Cephalexin?" This antibiotic has become a trusted solution for various bacterial infections, especially when the body needs a little extra help clearing out stubborn bugs. Let's explore some of the most common uses and how Cephalexin works in everyday scenarios.

One of the main reasons people end up with a Cephalexin prescription is for **skin infections**. Think of conditions like cellulitis, where bacteria sneak in through a small cut or scrape, causing redness, swelling, and warmth. Infections like this can spread quickly if left untreated, but with Cephalexin on board, the bacteria are stopped in their tracks, allowing the skin to heal before things get out of hand.

Respiratory infections are another area where Cephalexin comes to the rescue. Although it's not the first choice for conditions like sinusitis or bronchitis, it's often used when other antibiotics aren't an option. Picture an elderly patient with chronic bronchitis who's already tried a few rounds of antibiotics with little success—Cephalexin might be the one that finally does the trick.

Urinary tract infections (UTIs) are another common reason doctors reach for Cephalexin. Imagine an otherwise healthy adult who suddenly finds themselves running to the bathroom every hour, only to feel that frustrating burn with each trip. A few doses of Cephalexin can quickly bring relief by eliminating the bacteria causing the infection. While it's often used for simple UTIs, Cephalexin can also be prescribed to older patients or people with recurrent infections to help prevent further problems.

Beyond these, Cephalexin plays a critical role in treating **ear infections**, especially for children. If you've ever cared for a child with an ear infection, you know how miserable they can be—crying, tugging at their ear, and struggling to sleep. Cephalexin helps clear the bacteria in the middle ear, providing relief and reducing the chances of complications like hearing loss.

Dentists also rely on Cephalexin when infections crop up in unexpected places—like a painful abscess lurking around a tooth. Dental infections can get serious if they aren't dealt with quickly, but Cephalexin helps contain the infection, buying time until the dentist can perform any necessary procedures.

There's another important role Cephalexin plays: **preventative care**. Sometimes, doctors prescribe it as a preventive measure, such as before certain surgeries. For example, patients with joint replacements might take Cephalexin to lower the risk of infection during dental work or other procedures that could introduce bacteria into the bloodstream. This kind of prevention ensures small issues don't snowball into more serious infections.

While Cephalexin covers a lot of ground, it's essential to know that it's not a cure-all. It works best against specific bacteria, and it won't help with viral infections like the common cold or flu. Using it responsibly means following your doctor's instructions and not requesting antibiotics when they aren't needed—this helps prevent antibiotic resistance and keeps medications like Cephalexin effective for those who really need them.

Whether it's calming the pain of a UTI, soothing a child's aching ear, or preventing an infection after surgery, Cephalexin is a reliable option with a long track record of success. Each time it's used, it's playing a small but crucial role in helping people recover and stay well, making it a staple in both medicine cabinets and hospital pharmacies alike.

CHAPTER 2

When Is Cephalexin Prescribed?

You might wonder, "When exactly do doctors decide that Cephalexin is the right choice?" Understanding when and why this antibiotic is prescribed can give you a clearer picture of how it fits into everyday healthcare. Let's walk through some real-world examples where Cephalexin often plays a vital role, from minor infections to precautionary care.

Imagine this: a child returns from a weekend playing outside with a few scrapes on their knee. At first, it looks harmless, but by the next day, the area is red and swollen. The doctor diagnoses **cellulitis**, a bacterial infection that can spread if untreated. This is one of those moments when Cephalexin becomes essential—it helps stop the bacteria from multiplying and allows the child's immune system to take over and heal the wound. Similarly, Cephalexin is often prescribed for **respiratory infections**, though it's not always the first option. Let's say someone has been battling sinusitis for weeks, and the usual antibiotics don't seem to be working. Or maybe a person with chronic bronchitis develops an infection that complicates their condition. In such cases, Cephalexin steps in, offering a second line of defense to help clear the infection.

One of the more familiar scenarios involves **urinary tract infections** (UTIs). Anyone who has experienced the discomfort of a UTI knows how quickly it can turn a normal day into a miserable one. Imagine waking up, needing to visit the bathroom repeatedly, only to be greeted with burning pain each time. For simple UTIs, Cephalexin is often the go-to solution, easing symptoms and preventing the infection from traveling to the kidneys, where it could cause more serious issues.

Then, there's **ear infections**, particularly in children. Ear infections are a common reason for late-night trips to urgent care, with children in pain, pulling at their ears, and struggling to sleep. Cephalexin provides relief by targeting the bacteria in the middle ear, allowing the child to recover and return to their playful self within a few days.

Sometimes, doctors prescribe Cephalexin not just to treat infections but also to **prevent them**. Picture this: an elderly patient with an artificial knee scheduled for a routine dental cleaning. To minimize the risk of bacteria from the mouth traveling to the joint and causing an infection, the doctor may prescribe Cephalexin as a preventive measure. Similarly, it's used before certain surgeries to lower the chance of postoperative infections, helping patients recover smoothly.

In some cases, Cephalexin even makes an appearance in **dental care**. An untreated tooth infection can quickly become serious, with pain spreading to the jaw or even causing facial swelling. Dentists sometimes prescribe Cephalexin to manage these infections or prevent complications until further dental work can be done. It's important to remember, though, that Cephalexin isn't a catch-all remedy. It's effective against bacterial infections, but it won't work for viral illnesses like the flu or a common cold. Doctors use it with care, selecting it only when it's likely to be the most effective option.

Whether treating an infection or preventing one, Cephalexin remains a reliable tool in a doctor's kit. Each prescription serves a purpose, helping patients recover more quickly or avoid complications. It's these small but significant uses that make Cephalexin such a staple across different areas of medicine, offering peace of mind to patients and healthcare providers alike.

2.1 Treating Bacterial Infections

When it comes to treating bacterial infections, Cephalexin often plays a key role in getting patients back on their feet. Bacteria can sneak into the body in many ways—through a scrape on the skin, a sore throat, or even a simple dental procedure. Left unchecked, these infections can grow, causing pain, discomfort, or, in some cases, serious health risks. This is where antibiotics like Cephalexin come into the picture, working quietly but powerfully to help the body heal. You might wonder how a doctor decides that Cephalexin is the right fit for an infection. The answer lies in the kind of bacteria causing the problem. Cephalexin is a first-generation **cephalosporin**, meaning it's particularly effective against bacteria like *Staphylococcus* and *Streptococcus*—the usual suspects behind infections of the skin, throat, and urinary tract. So, when a doctor sees one of these culprits at work, Cephalexin is often prescribed to stop the bacteria in their tracks.

Let's take **skin infections** as an example. Imagine you nick yourself while gardening, and within a few days, the wound becomes red, warm, and swollen. What started as a minor scratch can quickly turn into cellulitis, a bacterial infection that spreads through the skin. Cephalexin is commonly prescribed to treat this kind of infection, helping to reduce the inflammation and prevent further spread.

Another everyday scenario involves **UTIs** (urinary tract infections). If you've ever had one, you know how unpleasant it can be—burning sensations, frequent bathroom trips, and a constant feeling of urgency. Cephalexin targets the bacteria responsible, offering relief and stopping the infection from reaching the kidneys, where it could cause more serious complications.

Cephalexin is also a familiar name in treating **respiratory infections** like sinusitis or bronchitis. When these infections are caused by bacteria and refuse to clear up on their own, Cephalexin helps the body fight off the invaders. It might not be the first option for every respiratory infection, but it serves as a reliable choice when other treatments fall short.

Doctors also turn to Cephalexin to manage **dental infections**. Imagine having a throbbing toothache caused by an infected tooth. Left untreated, the infection could spread to surrounding tissues or even enter the bloodstream. In such cases, Cephalexin is prescribed to control the infection until more permanent dental treatment, like a root canal or extraction, can be done. One of the reasons Cephalexin is so widely trusted is its predictable action—it's known to work well for common bacterial infections and typically has fewer side effects than more powerful antibiotics. That makes it an excellent option for patients who need effective treatment but don't require the "big guns" of antibiotic therapy. However, it's important to remember that Cephalexin only works on **bacterial infections**. If you or someone you know has a viral infection—like a cold or the flu—Cephalexin won't be helpful. Taking antibiotics unnecessarily not only won't help you feel better but can also contribute to **antibiotic resistance**, a growing global health concern.

In the right hands, though, Cephalexin offers a dependable way to treat infections, reduce symptoms, and speed up recovery. Whether it's a child with an ear infection or an adult with a stubborn UTI, Cephalexin is often part of the solution, ensuring that life can quickly return to normal.

2.2 Conditions It Covers (Respiratory, Skin, UTI, and More)

Cephalexin is a versatile antibiotic, used to treat a wide range of bacterial infections that can show up in different parts of the body. You might have heard of it being prescribed for things like respiratory infections or skin issues, but its usefulness extends even further.

Let's take a closer look at some of the most common conditions it covers—and why it's often the go-to choice in these situations. One of the most familiar uses is for **respiratory infections**. Imagine dealing with sinusitis or bronchitis that just won't go away—where symptoms like congestion, coughing, or a persistent headache make it hard to get through the day. When these infections are caused by bacteria, Cephalexin can step in to help clear things up. It's not the first choice for every respiratory issue, especially if the cause is viral, but when bacterial involvement is suspected, it becomes a helpful part of the treatment plan.

Skin infections are another area where Cephalexin shines. Picture a small cut or scrape that becomes swollen, red, and tender to the touch. It may start as something minor but can quickly turn into a more serious problem like cellulitis, where the infection spreads under the skin. Doctors often prescribe Cephalexin to tackle such infections early, preventing them from escalating into something more severe. For people prone to recurring skin infections, it's also a familiar ally.

Then there are **urinary tract infections** (UTIs), which can make even the simplest of days feel unbearable. If you've ever experienced one, you know that the constant urge to urinate, coupled with burning discomfort, can make it hard to focus on anything else. Cephalexin is frequently prescribed to treat UTIs, particularly in women and older adults who are more prone to these infections. It helps stop the bacteria responsible from spreading, providing relief and protecting the kidneys from further complications.

But Cephalexin's usefulness doesn't stop there. It also plays an important role in managing **bone infections** like osteomyelitis, as well as **dental infections**—especially when an infection flares up around a tooth before a procedure can be performed. For example, imagine a dental abscess causing severe pain just before a root canal. In such cases, Cephalexin helps control the infection until the underlying issue can be properly treated.

For people with weakened immune systems or certain medical conditions, infections can pose an even greater risk. Cephalexin is often used in these situations as a **preventive measure**, especially before surgeries or dental work, to reduce the chance of infection. This is particularly important for patients with joint replacements or heart conditions, where even a minor infection can become dangerous. Because Cephalexin covers such a broad spectrum of bacterial infections, it's a medication that people of all ages—whether children, adults, or seniors—may encounter at some point. The key is using it correctly and only when it's truly needed. Taking it without a real bacterial infection won't help and could even make things worse in the long run by contributing to antibiotic resistance.

Whether it's calming an irritated sinus, soothing an infected wound, or relieving the discomfort of a UTI, Cephalexin plays an important role in helping people recover and get back to their routines. Its flexibility and reliability have earned it a trusted spot on doctors' prescription pads—and for good reason.

2.3 Who Should and Shouldn't Use Cephalexin

Cephalexin can be incredibly effective, but it's not the right solution for everyone. Just like any medication, it works best when prescribed for the right people under the right circumstances. So, who should use Cephalexin, and who might need to steer clear of it? Let's break it down in a simple, relatable way.

You might be wondering if Cephalexin is suitable for you or a family member. It's most often prescribed to **children, adults, and seniors** dealing with bacterial infections like respiratory infections, skin issues, or UTIs. It's also useful for patients with weakened immune systems—like those undergoing chemotherapy or with chronic illnesses—who need extra protection from infections. In these cases, Cephalexin plays a role in both treating infections and sometimes preventing them from happening in the first place.

However, not everyone can use Cephalexin safely. If you or someone you know has **allergies to penicillin or other beta-lactam antibiotics**, there's a chance

Cephalexin could trigger an allergic reaction. For some, the symptoms may be mild—like a rash or itching—but for others, it could be more serious, leading to swelling or difficulty breathing. If you've ever had a bad reaction to antibiotics, it's essential to let your doctor know before starting Cephalexin.

Another group that should be cautious includes people with **kidney problems**. Cephalexin is processed through the kidneys, and if those organs aren't functioning well, the medication could build up in the body and cause unwanted side effects. Doctors may adjust the dose or choose a different antibiotic altogether to avoid complications.

Pregnant and breastfeeding women often ask if Cephalexin is safe. Generally, it's considered safe to use during pregnancy and while nursing, but it's still a good idea to discuss it with your doctor. For example, if a pregnant woman develops a UTI, Cephalexin might be prescribed because the benefits outweigh any potential risks. However, medical professionals always evaluate these situations carefully to make sure it's the right choice.

On the flip side, there are also cases where people take antibiotics when they shouldn't. For example, it's not uncommon for someone to think an antibiotic will help with a **cold or the flu**, only to learn later that these illnesses are caused by viruses, not bacteria. Antibiotics like Cephalexin won't help in these situations and could contribute to the growing problem of antibiotic resistance, making it harder to treat infections down the road. It's also important to avoid taking leftover Cephalexin from a previous illness or borrowing it from someone else.

You might feel tempted to take a few pills if symptoms feel familiar, but using the wrong antibiotic—or not completing the full prescribed course—can do more harm than good. Each infection is different, and doctors choose medications based on the specific bacteria involved.

So, who shouldn't use Cephalexin? People with known allergies to cephalosporins or penicillin need to avoid it, as do those with serious kidney problems unless closely monitored by a doctor. And it's a no-go for viral infections like colds or flu—save it for when bacteria are truly the culprit.

Ultimately, Cephalexin can be a powerful ally for the right patient at the right time. If prescribed appropriately and taken correctly, it helps patients recover quickly and keeps infections from spreading or worsening. But as with any medication, it's all about knowing when it's needed and when it's not, making sure the right people benefit while others avoid unnecessary risks. If you ever have doubts about whether Cephalexin is the right choice for you or a loved one, a quick conversation with your doctor can offer clarity and peace of mind.

CHAPTER 3

How to Take Cephalexin Safely

Taking medication might seem straightforward, but doing it safely is key to getting better and avoiding complications. Cephalexin, like any antibiotic, works best when taken correctly. In this chapter, we'll explore the essentials for using Cephalexin effectively, with some real-life examples and practical advice along the way.

You might wonder, "Does it matter if I take it before or after meals?" In general, Cephalexin can be taken with or without food, but many people find it's easier on the stomach if taken after a meal. A light snack or even a glass of milk can help reduce the chance of nausea, especially for kids or those prone to digestive issues. It's also important to **stick to a schedule**.

Antibiotics work best when they're taken at regular intervals, which helps maintain a steady level of the medication in your body. If you're supposed to take it every eight hours, setting alarms on your phone can be a lifesaver—especially if you're juggling work, kids, or other responsibilities. Missing doses or taking them at irregular times can weaken the medication's effectiveness, giving bacteria a chance to fight back.

If you've ever had to convince a child to take medicine, you know it can be a struggle. Cephalexin comes in both capsules and liquid form, making it easier for young ones or those who can't swallow pills. Some parents say mixing the liquid version with a bit of applesauce or juice makes the process smoother. Just be sure to use the provided measuring tool—eyeballing doses isn't safe, even if it feels close enough.

A common question is, "What if I miss a dose?" If that happens, the best approach is to take the missed dose as soon as you remember—unless it's almost time for the next one. In that case, skip the missed dose and stick to your schedule. Doubling up isn't a good idea, as it can increase the risk of side effects without any added benefit. And speaking of side effects, let's talk about **what to watch for**. While Cephalexin is generally well-tolerated, some people experience mild side effects like diarrhea or stomach discomfort. If the diarrhea becomes severe or contains blood, it's time to call the doctor. Rarely, an allergic reaction can occur, with symptoms like rash, itching, or trouble breathing. If that happens, seek medical attention immediately—it's better to be safe than sorry.

One of the most important things to remember is **finishing the full course of antibiotics**, even if you start to feel better halfway through. It can be tempting to stop when the symptoms improve, but doing so might leave some bacteria behind, allowing the infection to come back stronger. Think of it like cleaning a messy room—if you stop halfway, the clutter just piles up again.

Also, avoid sharing your prescription with others. It might seem helpful to pass along leftover pills to someone with similar symptoms, but this can backfire. The person might need a different antibiotic, or they could have an allergic reaction without knowing it. Each infection is unique, and only a doctor can determine the right medication and dosage. Another tip: **stay hydrated**. Drinking plenty of water helps your body process the medication and can also ease any mild side effects. It's a small habit that goes a long way in keeping things running smoothly while you recover.

Finally, always store Cephalexin properly. The capsules should be kept at room temperature, away from moisture and heat. If you have the liquid version, it needs to be refrigerated and used within the time frame your doctor or pharmacist provides. Taking expired medication isn't safe, even if it looks and smells fine. By following these simple steps, you'll give Cephalexin the best chance to do its job and help you feel better quickly. And if any questions or concerns pop up along the way, never hesitate to reach out to your healthcare provider. They're there to guide you, ensuring that you're on the right path to recovery.

3.1 Dosage Guidelines for Adults and Children

When it comes to taking antibiotics like Cephalexin, getting the dosage right is crucial. Too little, and the medication might not work as intended. Too much, and you could end up dealing with unnecessary side effects. In this section, we'll walk through the typical dosages for both adults and children, giving you a clearer idea of what to expect.

Let's start with adults. For most infections, the standard dose is **250 mg to 500 mg every six to twelve hours**. You might wonder, "Why is there a range?" Well, it all depends on the type and severity of the infection. For something like a mild skin infection, a lower dose might do the trick. But for tougher infections, like pneumonia or a serious urinary tract infection (UTI), the doctor might prescribe the higher end of the dosage range.

Now, let's talk about children. Dosing for kids isn't as straightforward since it's based on weight. In general, pediatric doses are **25 to 50 mg per kilogram of body weight per day**, divided into multiple doses. For example, if your child weighs 20 kilograms (around 44 pounds), the doctor might recommend a total daily dose of 500 to 1000 mg, spread out across several doses. It's a bit like splitting up a pie so everyone gets a fair share—you don't want to serve too much at once, but you also don't want to leave anyone hungry.

Parents might be familiar with the liquid version of Cephalexin, which is commonly used for children. If you've ever struggled to get a child to take medicine, you know it's no easy feat. Some parents swear by mixing the liquid with yogurt or juice to mask the taste. Just make sure you use the provided measuring spoon or syringe—using a kitchen spoon can lead to dosing mistakes.

You might wonder, "What if my child refuses to take the medicine?" This is more common than you'd think. One trick is to offer a small reward after they take it, like a sticker or extra screen time. It's also helpful to stay calm and patient. Kids can sense frustration, and if they see you're stressed, they might resist even more.

For both adults and children, consistency is key. Taking the medication at the same time every day makes it easier to remember and helps maintain steady levels of the drug in the body. If you or your child miss a dose, take it as soon as you remember—unless it's almost time for the next one. In that case, skip the missed dose to avoid doubling up.

People often ask if it's okay to stop taking Cephalexin once they start feeling better. This is a common mistake. Even if symptoms improve after a few days, it's important to finish the full course of antibiotics. Think of it like a relay race—if you stop running before the finish line, you won't complete the race, and the infection might come back stronger than before.

Of course, everyone's situation is unique, and dosages can vary based on factors like the type of infection, medical history, and other medications being taken. This is why it's essential to follow your doctor's instructions and ask questions if anything feels unclear.

If you're ever unsure about your dose or how to give the medicine to a child, don't hesitate to call your healthcare provider or pharmacist. They've seen it all and are there to help, whether you're dealing with a stubborn toddler or trying to keep track of your own medication schedule. After all, getting the dosage right is one of the easiest ways to make sure Cephalexin does its job and helps you get back on your feet.

3.2 What to Expect During Treatment

Starting a course of Cephalexin can feel like a relief, especially if you've been dealing with a nagging infection. But you might wonder, "What will the next few days look like? How will I know it's working?" Understanding what to expect during treatment can make the process smoother and ease any worries you may have.

For most people, relief begins within **48 to 72 hours** of starting the medication. If you're treating something like a urinary tract infection (UTI), you might notice that the burning sensation when you pee starts to fade, and those frequent trips to the bathroom slow down. Similarly, if you've been struggling with a sinus infection, you may wake up one morning and realize you can breathe through your nose again.

But it's not always an instant fix. Some infections, especially deeper ones like respiratory or skin infections, might take longer to show improvement. This doesn't mean the antibiotic isn't working—just that your body needs time to heal.

During treatment, you may also experience mild side effects. A common one is **stomach discomfort**. You might notice some nausea, mild diarrhea, or even a bit of bloating. This is normal since antibiotics can disrupt the balance of good and bad bacteria in your gut. To help, you could try eating small meals or adding probiotics like yogurt to your diet, which some people find soothing.

Another question that pops up is, "Will I feel tired while on Cephalexin?" While the medication itself doesn't cause drowsiness, fighting an infection can drain your energy. It's your body's way of asking for rest, so listen to it. Taking naps or going to bed a little earlier might be just what you need. On the other hand, there are things to watch out for. **Allergic reactions**, while uncommon, can happen. If you notice a rash, itching, or swelling, it's important to contact your doctor. Severe reactions like difficulty breathing are rare but require immediate medical attention.

People also wonder, "Can I drink alcohol while taking Cephalexin?" While there's no strict rule against it, drinking alcohol might make the side effects—like stomach discomfort—feel worse. If you can, it's best to take a break from alcohol until you finish your course of antibiotics. Your body will thank you. If you're treating a child, it helps to know that kids can sometimes become a bit cranky or restless during treatment. This isn't unusual. Antibiotics can mess with their little routines, especially if side effects like an upset tummy kick in. Keep communication open—offering comfort, extra snuggles, and some quiet time with their favorite activities can make the process less stressful for both of you.

One of the most important things during treatment is **completing the full course**, even if you feel better halfway through. Think of it like scrubbing a stain out of fabric—if you stop too soon, some of it lingers and could spread again. Skipping doses or ending the medication early might allow the infection to come back, potentially stronger than before.

It's also helpful to know what happens when the treatment ends. For many, life returns to normal without a hitch. However, if symptoms linger or return after completing the course, it's essential to call your doctor. Sometimes, infections need a bit more time or a different approach. Taking Cephalexin is a bit like following a trusted map—you know where you're headed, but the journey might have a few bumps along the way. With some patience, proper care, and an open line of communication with your healthcare provider, you'll be on the road to recovery in no time. And remember, it's okay to ask questions or reach out if something feels off—your health is always worth the extra attention.

3.3 Importance of Completing the Course

You're a few days into your Cephalexin treatment, and things are finally looking up. The symptoms that made you feel miserable are starting to ease. Naturally, you might wonder, "Do I really need to finish the whole course? I feel better already!" It's tempting to stop early, but completing your full antibiotic course is one of the most important steps toward a complete recovery. Let's explore why that's the case.

Imagine washing a dirty plate with dried food stuck on it. You scrub the surface, and it looks clean after a few moments, but if you stop too soon, those tough little spots you missed can still cling on. The same logic applies to infections. Cephalexin begins working quickly, wiping out many bacteria in the first few days. But some of the more stubborn bacteria might still be hanging around, just waiting for the perfect moment to bounce back if you stop taking the medicine too soon.

When that happens, not only can the infection return, but it might come back stronger. You might have heard of antibiotic resistance—a growing concern where bacteria learn to outsmart antibiotics. If you don't complete the course, you give these bacteria a chance to adapt and become tougher to treat the next time around. And that's when simple infections can turn into complicated ones, requiring more aggressive medications or longer treatments.

Many people stop their antibiotics early simply because they feel better. It's a common reaction—who wouldn't want to skip a few doses if the worst seems to be over? But this is where antibiotics differ from pain relievers or cold medicine. Even when you start feeling fine, the infection hasn't completely disappeared. Cephalexin needs time to finish the job and ensure every last bacterium is gone. Think of it as a marathon rather than a sprint—crossing the finish line is just as important as how fast you run.

Children can also be a challenge when it comes to finishing a prescription. Maybe your child's ear infection seems better, and they're tired of taking that medicine that tastes, well, not great. It's easy to understand the struggle, but skipping doses can lead to lingering infections, meaning another round of medication or even a return trip to the doctor's office. A little creativity—like offering a sticker after every dose or mixing the medicine with a favorite snack—can go a long way in ensuring they complete the course.

You might also find yourself wondering, "What if I forget a dose?" Life gets busy, and missing a pill here or there happens to the best of us. The key is not to panic. If you remember soon after the scheduled time, take the dose as soon as possible. If it's almost time for your next dose, though, just skip the missed one—doubling up isn't recommended, as it could cause more side effects. And let's not forget the satisfaction of knowing you've done everything in your power to recover fully.

Completing the course means fewer chances of complications down the road. You can move on with life without worrying about that infection sneaking back when you least expect it. Finishing a course of antibiotics isn't just about your own health, either—it's about the bigger picture. By taking antibiotics responsibly, you play a small but meaningful role in preventing the spread of antibiotic resistance, helping ensure that these medications will work for others in the future.

In the end, think of it this way: completing the full course is an investment in your well-being. You've already come this far, and a few more days of pills or capsules are worth the peace of mind that comes with knowing you've taken every step toward recovery. Your future self will thank you.

CHAPTER 4

Potential Side Effects and Risks

When starting any medication, it's natural to wonder, "What if something goes wrong?" Cephalexin, like many antibiotics, can come with its own set of side effects. The good news is that most people tolerate it well, but it's still important to know what to expect, just in case. Understanding the potential risks allows you to stay calm and handle any reactions that might come up.

One of the most common side effects people experience with Cephalexin is mild stomach upset. This might feel like a bit of nausea, or you may notice loose stools. Imagine you've just eaten something a little too rich for dinner—your stomach grumbles, and you spend some extra time in the bathroom. It's annoying, but usually nothing to worry about. Taking Cephalexin with food often helps reduce these digestive issues, so try pairing it with meals to make things easier on your stomach.

Another minor side effect can be a headache or a bit of dizziness. You know that feeling when you get up too fast and everything spins for a second? It's not exactly pleasant, but it usually passes quickly. If you find yourself feeling lightheaded on Cephalexin, it's a good idea to stay hydrated and avoid sudden movements until your body adjusts.

Some people also report itching or a mild skin rash. These symptoms can be tricky since they might make you wonder, "Is this just a harmless reaction, or something more serious?" If the itching is mild and goes away on its own, it's usually nothing alarming. However, if the rash spreads, becomes severe, or is accompanied by swelling or difficulty breathing, it could be an allergic reaction. In that case, it's essential to stop taking the medication and contact your doctor right away. Allergic reactions to Cephalexin are rare but can happen, especially in people with penicillin allergies.

There's also the possibility of yeast infections, especially for women. Antibiotics, while great at killing harmful bacteria, can sometimes disrupt the natural balance of good bacteria in the body, leading to infections like thrush. If you notice itching, discharge, or other signs of a yeast infection during or after treatment, it's worth bringing it up with your doctor. They may recommend a probiotic or antifungal treatment to restore balance.

In rare cases, Cephalexin can cause more serious side effects, like severe diarrhea. If you experience frequent, watery stools, especially with blood or mucus, it could be a sign of a condition called *Clostridium difficile* infection (or *C. diff* for short). Though uncommon, this type of diarrhea can happen when antibiotics disrupt the gut's natural bacteria too much. If this happens, don't hesitate to reach out to your healthcare provider. They can offer guidance on how to manage it and determine if you need further treatment.

You might also wonder if Cephalexin affects your liver or kidneys, and the answer is—only in very rare cases. People with pre-existing liver or kidney conditions should be monitored closely, but for most healthy individuals, there's little cause for concern. If you notice unusual symptoms like dark urine, yellowing of the skin or eyes, or extreme fatigue, those could be signs of a problem worth mentioning to your doctor.

It's also good to know that mixing alcohol with Cephalexin doesn't usually cause serious interactions, though drinking in moderation is always a wise choice. Heavy drinking could irritate your stomach further or make side effects like dizziness worse. If you're planning a celebratory dinner while on antibiotics, a glass of wine probably won't hurt, but it's still a good idea to stay mindful of how your body feels.

The bottom line is this: while side effects are possible, most people who take Cephalexin experience only mild, manageable symptoms—if any at all. Listening to your body is the best approach. If something doesn't feel right, reach out to your healthcare provider. They can help you figure out whether what you're experiencing is part of the normal course or if adjustments need to be made.

Remember, taking care of yourself means staying informed, but it also means not worrying too much about every "what if." By knowing what to expect and how to respond, you'll be prepared for a smooth and safe treatment experience.

4.1 Common Side Effects

When taking any medication, it's natural to wonder, "Is this going to make me feel off?" With Cephalexin, most people do just fine, but it's good to know what side effects might come along. The good news is that the most common side effects are mild and manageable, often disappearing on their own as your body adjusts. Let's walk through some of the ones you might encounter so that you know what's normal—and when to call your doctor.

A little upset stomach is probably the most common side effect. You know that gurgly, uneasy feeling you sometimes get after eating too much spicy food? That's a pretty close comparison. Cephalexin can cause some nausea, mild stomach cramps, or loose stools, especially early in the treatment. Taking your dose with food is usually all it takes to keep your stomach happy. If you forget and take it on an empty stomach, don't worry—you might just feel a little queasy for a while.

Diarrhea is also something people sometimes notice while on antibiotics. Think of it like your body saying, "Hey, we're clearing things out here." While this can be annoying, it's usually temporary. If it's mild, just make sure you drink plenty of fluids to stay hydrated. But if diarrhea becomes severe or lasts too long, it's worth checking in with your doctor. Another thing that can come up is a headache. You know those dull, nagging headaches that come on after a long day of staring at screens? Cephalexin headaches are usually similar—they're not intense but can be a bit of a nuisance. Staying well-hydrated and resting when you can should help ease the discomfort. If you're already prone to headaches, it might be a good idea to have some over-the-counter pain relief handy.

Some people also experience a bit of dizziness, like that lightheaded sensation when you stand up too quickly. It's not super common, but if it happens to you, try to take it easy. Sitting or lying down for a few minutes should help. If you're planning to drive or operate machinery, it's probably best to wait until you know how your body reacts to the medication.

Skin reactions like mild rashes or itching are possible, though not very common. If you notice a little redness or itchiness, it could just be your body adjusting to the medication. However, if the rash becomes widespread or you start experiencing swelling or difficulty breathing, that's a sign you might be having an allergic reaction, and you'll want to contact your doctor immediately.

Yeast infections are another side effect that can happen, especially for women. Antibiotics can sometimes upset the balance of good bacteria in the body, leading to issues like thrush or vaginal yeast infections. If you notice itching, unusual discharge, or discomfort, talk to your healthcare provider. They may suggest a probiotic or antifungal treatment to keep things in balance.

While these side effects might sound like a lot, it's important to remember that most people don't experience all of them—and some won't experience any at all. The key is to listen to your body. If something feels off, don't hesitate to ask your healthcare provider. It's always better to get a little peace of mind than to worry unnecessarily. And here's a comforting thought: Many people take Cephalexin without any side effects at all. The ones that do occur are typically minor and temporary, clearing up as your body gets used to the medication. Just remember, your body is working hard to heal—and sometimes that comes with a few bumps along the way.

4.2 Recognizing Allergic Reactions

Taking a new medication can sometimes feel a little nerve-wracking, especially if you've heard about the possibility of allergic reactions. If you're starting Cephalexin, you might wonder, "What if I'm allergic to it?" The good news is that most people tolerate the medication just fine, but it's important to know what to watch for, just in case. Recognizing the signs early can make a big difference.

Allergic reactions can show up in different ways, ranging from mild symptoms like a skin rash to more serious situations that require medical attention. Let's start with the mild ones, which are more common. Imagine you've just taken your first few doses, and suddenly you notice an itchy red rash. This might seem like no big deal—it could just be your body adjusting. But if the rash spreads or gets worse, it's worth giving your doctor a call to be on the safe side.

Hives are another sign to keep in mind. They appear as raised, itchy bumps on the skin, sometimes looking a bit like mosquito bites. If you've ever broken out in hives after eating certain foods, the reaction to Cephalexin might feel familiar. Again, a mild rash or a few hives might not be urgent, but they're worth monitoring. Things get more serious if other symptoms start to show up, like swelling—especially around the lips, eyes, or throat. This could signal a more intense allergic response called angioedema. Imagine feeling fine one moment, and the next, your face feels puffy or your throat starts to feel tight. That's a sign you need to seek medical help right away.

Breathing issues are another red flag. If you start wheezing or feel like it's harder to catch your breath, it's time to act quickly. These symptoms can point to anaphylaxis, a rare but dangerous reaction that requires immediate care. Think of it like your body pressing the emergency brake—it needs help fast. Sometimes, allergic reactions can sneak up on you. You might feel lightheaded or experience nausea, which could be your body's way of saying, "Something isn't right here." While these symptoms alone aren't always linked to a serious allergy, it's good to pay attention to what your body is telling you. If something feels off—whether it's a racing heart or unexpected swelling—it's always better to err on the side of caution.

Here's a comforting thought: Serious allergic reactions to Cephalexin are quite rare. Most people who develop a mild rash or other minor symptoms will recover quickly without complications. However, knowing what to look for can help you act early and avoid anything more serious.

If you've had allergic reactions to antibiotics like penicillin in the past, it's a good idea to mention it to your doctor before starting Cephalexin. There's a small chance of cross-reactivity between these two medications, meaning that people allergic to penicillin might have a similar reaction to Cephalexin. But don't worry—there are plenty of other antibiotic options if that's the case.

In the end, the key takeaway is this: listen to your body. If you notice anything unusual, even if it seems small, reach out to your healthcare provider. They can guide you on whether you need to stop the medication or adjust your treatment plan. And remember, most people complete their course of Cephalexin without a hitch. But having the knowledge to recognize allergic reactions gives you peace of mind—and that's always worth having.

4.3 When to Contact a Doctor

Taking a medication like Cephalexin often goes smoothly, but every now and then, things can feel a bit off. You might wonder, "Is this side effect normal, or should I call my doctor?" It's a great question—and knowing when to reach out can make all the difference. Let's walk through some scenarios that might pop up during your treatment and help you decide when it's time to seek medical advice.

First, let's talk about the not-so-scary stuff. Mild side effects like a little nausea or an upset stomach aren't uncommon. Maybe you take Cephalexin with breakfast, and a couple of hours later, you feel a bit queasy. In most cases, this kind of discomfort isn't something to stress over. A snack with your next dose or plenty of water might be all you need to feel better. But if the nausea becomes persistent or you start vomiting, that's your body saying it might need extra help—definitely a good reason to call your doctor.

Now, imagine you've been on Cephalexin for a few days and suddenly develop a rash. A small, itchy patch might not be urgent, but if the rash spreads quickly or is accompanied by swelling, it's time to pay attention. This could be a sign of an allergic reaction. Even if you feel okay otherwise, it's smart to reach out to your healthcare provider before the symptoms escalate.

Speaking of swelling, if you notice any puffiness around your lips, face, or throat, don't wait—this can point to a serious reaction called angioedema. And if you find yourself wheezing or struggling to breathe, head to the emergency room immediately. It's rare, but allergic reactions like these can progress quickly, and it's better to get help fast than take any chances.

Another scenario to watch for is diarrhea. It might seem like no big deal at first—maybe just a side effect, right? But if the diarrhea is severe or comes with stomach cramps or blood, it could be a sign of a more serious issue like *Clostridium difficile* (C. diff) infection, which sometimes happens after taking antibiotics. If that happens, don't hesitate to contact your doctor.

Also, pay attention to how you're feeling overall. Cephalexin is supposed to help you feel better, so if you notice no improvement after a few days—or if your symptoms get worse—it's a good idea to check in with your doctor. For example, if you're taking it for a UTI and still feel burning or pain when you urinate, it might mean the bacteria causing the infection is resistant to the medication, and your treatment plan needs adjusting.

Another red flag to look out for is sudden fatigue or dizziness. If you find yourself feeling unusually tired or lightheaded, especially alongside other symptoms like fever or shortness of breath, this could point to something more serious that requires medical attention. Parents, if your child is taking Cephalexin and seems fussier than usual, develops a fever, or refuses to eat or drink, don't hesitate to call the pediatrician. Kids can't always explain what's wrong, so trust your gut if something feels off.

Lastly, if you're dealing with any other chronic conditions—like kidney problems or diabetes—and notice a change in your health during treatment, it's a good idea to check in. Even if it seems unrelated, certain symptoms might signal an interaction between Cephalexin and your other medications.

In short, you know your body (or your child's) best. If something feels unusual or makes you uncomfortable, trust that instinct and reach out to your healthcare provider. It's better to ask and be reassured than to wait and wonder. Most of the time, your doctor can easily adjust your dosage or recommend ways to manage side effects. And remember, the goal is to feel better—so don't hesitate to get the support you need along the way.

CHAPTER 5

Drug Interactions and Precautions

When you're taking a medication like Cephalexin, it's easy to assume you can just follow the instructions and be on your way. But here's the thing: medications don't exist in a bubble. They interact with other drugs, supplements, or even certain foods. Knowing what to watch for can make a huge difference in staying safe and getting the best results from your treatment. This chapter will walk you through some key interactions and precautions, so you can feel more confident about what to avoid and how to manage your health while on Cephalexin.

You might wonder, "Why would one medication affect another?" Well, imagine your body is like a busy airport. Medications act like planes, and each one needs clearance to land and do its job. If too many arrive at the same time—or if the air traffic controllers aren't communicating—things can get messy. Some drugs might block others from working properly, while others can intensify side effects, making you feel worse than the condition you're treating.

For example, if you're taking blood thinners like warfarin, Cephalexin can increase the risk of bleeding. It's not something that happens to everyone, but it's good to keep an eye out for signs like easy bruising or bleeding gums. In these cases, your doctor might adjust the dose of your blood thinner to keep everything running smoothly. Then there's the matter of birth control pills. You might have heard that antibiotics can make birth control less effective. While this interaction isn't as common as people think, it's still worth being cautious. If you're on hormonal contraception, ask your doctor whether you need a backup method like condoms while taking Cephalexin—better safe than sorry.

Certain diuretics, or "water pills," can also interfere with how Cephalexin works, especially if you're on them for high blood pressure. Diuretics increase urination, which can alter how quickly your body processes antibiotics. If you're taking both, it's worth a quick conversation with your doctor to ensure your medication schedule is balanced. If you're into vitamins or herbal supplements, don't forget that they count, too. Some supplements—like calcium, magnesium, or iron—can interfere with the absorption of antibiotics, including Cephalexin. A practical tip is to avoid taking these supplements at the same time as your antibiotic. For example, if you usually take your vitamins in the morning, try spacing them out by a few hours or taking Cephalexin at a different time of day.

Alcohol is another thing people often ask about. While Cephalexin doesn't have a severe interaction with alcohol, drinking too much can still weaken your immune system, making it harder for your body to fight off the infection. It can also increase the likelihood of side effects like nausea or dizziness. So, it's a good idea to go easy on alcohol while you're on antibiotics—your body will thank you for it.

You might also need to take some precautions if you have existing health conditions. For instance, people with kidney problems need to be careful, as their bodies may not filter Cephalexin as efficiently. If this applies to you, your doctor may adjust the dosage or suggest regular monitoring to make sure the medication is working without overloading your system.

Finally, if you're caring for an older adult or a child on Cephalexin, it's essential to keep an eye on how they're responding to the treatment. Kids and seniors are more sensitive to drug interactions, so be sure to share all their medications, including over-the-counter ones, with their doctor. Something as simple as a cold remedy or allergy medication can sometimes cause unexpected interactions.

In the end, managing medications isn't about being paranoid—it's about being prepared. If you're ever unsure whether something you're taking will interact with Cephalexin, just ask. Your pharmacist or healthcare provider is there to help, and they've likely seen similar situations before. A quick phone call can prevent complications and make sure you're getting the most from your treatment.

By staying mindful of potential interactions and following a few simple precautions, you'll be on your way to recovery without unnecessary bumps along the way. And remember, if something doesn't feel right—like a new symptom that catches you off guard—reach out to your doctor. It's always better to ask questions than to take risks with your health.

5.1 Medications That May Interact with Cephalexin

When you're prescribed Cephalexin, it's easy to think it's a simple fix for an infection. But here's the reality: medications can sometimes play a complicated game of tug-of-war with each other. Just like in a team sport, if one player isn't doing their job or gets sidelined, it can affect the entire game. In this section, we'll dive into some common medications that might interact with Cephalexin and what you should keep in mind to stay healthy.

You might wonder, "What types of medications should I be worried about?" Let's start with some everyday examples. If you're on blood thinners, such as warfarin, you need to tread carefully. Cephalexin can increase the effectiveness of these medications, raising your risk of bleeding. Imagine if you cut your finger while chopping veggies; it could bleed more than usual. That's not the scenario anyone wants. If you're on warfarin and get prescribed Cephalexin, it's crucial to communicate with your healthcare provider. They may adjust your blood thinner dose or keep an eye on your INR (International Normalized Ratio) levels to ensure everything stays in check.

Then there are antacids, particularly those that contain magnesium or aluminum. You know those chewy tablets that help settle your stomach after a spicy meal? They can interfere with how well Cephalexin is absorbed by your body. If you take both, try to space them out by at least a couple of hours. Picture this: you're trying to fill a glass with water, but someone keeps splashing it everywhere. That's what antacids can do to your antibiotic—making it harder for your body to soak up all the good stuff.

If you're taking certain diuretics, or "water pills," be cautious too. They can alter how your body processes Cephalexin, potentially affecting its efficacy. Think of diuretics as those pesky traffic lights that can hold up a long line of cars. If you're on a diuretic, your doctor may want to monitor how your body responds to Cephalexin to make sure everything flows smoothly. And let's not forget about hormonal contraceptives. There's a common myth that antibiotics always reduce the effectiveness of birth control pills. While this isn't true for Cephalexin specifically, it's still wise to ask your doctor or pharmacist about it. You don't want any surprises if you're relying on those pills for family planning.

You might also need to be careful if you're taking certain antifungals or medications for seizures. These can potentially interact with Cephalexin, leading to unwanted side effects or reduced effectiveness. Imagine your body as a symphony orchestra; if one musician is out of sync, it can throw off the entire performance.

If you're on any over-the-counter medications, like ibuprofen or other NSAIDs (nonsteroidal anti-inflammatory drugs), keep in mind that these can increase the risk of kidney issues when combined with Cephalexin, especially if you're already dealing with dehydration or existing kidney problems. It's like trying to juggle too many balls at once; eventually, something might drop.

So, what's the best approach? Communication is key. Don't hesitate to reach out to your healthcare provider or pharmacist if you're unsure about any potential interactions. They're there to help and can provide valuable insights tailored to your specific situation. And remember to keep a list of all the medications, vitamins, and supplements you're taking, as this can make conversations with your healthcare provider much smoother.

Ultimately, being proactive about understanding medication interactions can make a big difference in your treatment experience. It's not about being overly cautious but about being smart and informed. By knowing which medications may interact with Cephalexin, you can ensure that you're getting the most effective treatment while minimizing any risks. So stay curious, ask questions, and take charge of your health—you're the best advocate for your own well-being.

5.2 Impact of Alcohol and Food on Effectiveness

When you're taking medication like Cephalexin, it's easy to think that popping a pill is all there is to it. But the truth is, what you eat and drink can significantly affect how well that medication works. You might be wondering, "Can I enjoy my favorite meal or have a drink while I'm on this antibiotic?" Let's dive into the details so you can make informed choices.

First off, let's talk about food. Many people worry about whether to take medication on an empty stomach or with food. For Cephalexin, it's generally safe to take it with or without food. However, if you find that it upsets your stomach, having it with a meal can help ease any discomfort. Imagine your stomach as a busy kitchen; sometimes, when too much is happening at once, it can get a little chaotic. Having food in your system might help calm things down.

But there are some foods you might want to keep an eye on. Dairy products, like milk or cheese, can interfere with the absorption of certain antibiotics, although this isn't a significant issue with Cephalexin.

If you've ever seen a recipe where certain ingredients clash, it's a bit like that. While a splash of milk in your coffee can be delightful, mixing too much dairy right before taking your medication isn't the best idea. If you're going to enjoy dairy, aim for a couple of hours before or after taking your antibiotic.

You might also be curious about how alcohol fits into the picture. While it might seem harmless to have a glass of wine or a beer, mixing alcohol with antibiotics is often discouraged. Many people worry that alcohol can reduce the effectiveness of their medication. In the case of Cephalexin, moderate alcohol consumption is generally considered safe, but it can still lead to some unwanted side effects.

Think about it this way: if you're out celebrating and enjoying a drink, the last thing you want is to feel nauseous or dizzy because of a bad mix. Alcohol can also put extra stress on your liver, which is already busy processing the medication. So, if you choose to indulge, moderation is key. You might have heard stories from friends or family who had a rough experience mixing alcohol and antibiotics. Perhaps they felt tired or had a headache the next day. It's these personal anecdotes that make the connection clear: while it's not a strict no-go with Cephalexin, being mindful of your alcohol intake can make your treatment smoother.

Additionally, consider your overall health and any other medications you might be taking. If you're on medication for other conditions, like blood pressure or diabetes, adding alcohol into the mix could complicate things further. You wouldn't want to add extra ingredients to a recipe that's already challenging, right? Always consult with your healthcare provider if you're unsure.

In summary, while you can generally enjoy food and drink while taking Cephalexin, being cautious can enhance your treatment experience. Focus on balanced meals, keep an eye on dairy, and consider moderating your alcohol consumption. You want to give your body the best chance to heal, and making mindful choices about what you eat and drink can help you do just that. Your health is a team effort, and understanding how your lifestyle interacts with your medication is an important part of the game.

5.3 Managing Pre-Existing Conditions

When it comes to taking medications like Cephalexin, managing pre-existing conditions can feel like navigating a maze. You might wonder, "How does my asthma affect my treatment?" or "What about my diabetes?" These are common concerns, and understanding how your health history plays a role can make a big difference in your recovery journey.

Let's start with the basics. Pre-existing conditions are any health issues you had before starting a new medication. Think of them as little puzzle pieces in your health picture. When you're prescribed an antibiotic like Cephalexin, it's important to consider how these pieces fit together. For instance, if you have asthma, you might be concerned about whether taking an antibiotic could trigger an asthma attack.

Imagine a child with a recurring ear infection. Their doctor prescribes Cephalexin to help clear up the infection. But this child also has asthma. It's crucial for the parents to discuss the child's asthma history with the doctor. This ensures that the medication doesn't interfere with their asthma treatment. In most cases, Cephalexin doesn't affect asthma directly, but the added stress of an illness can sometimes provoke asthma symptoms. You might also have conditions like diabetes that require close attention when you're on medication. Antibiotics can sometimes alter blood sugar levels.

For example, if you're managing your blood sugar through diet and medication, taking Cephalexin might cause fluctuations. A person managing diabetes may notice their blood sugar levels dip unexpectedly. This is where communication with your healthcare provider becomes vital. They can offer strategies to monitor your levels more closely during your treatment.

Many people worry about the interactions between their medications for chronic conditions and the antibiotics they're taking. If you're on multiple prescriptions, such as blood thinners or medications for heart issues, it's important to have an open dialogue with your doctor. They can help identify any potential conflicts. Picture yourself at a dinner party where everyone is trying to talk at once; if you don't take a moment to listen and clarify, it can get confusing. The same goes for your medications—understanding how they work together is key.

Let's also talk about allergies. If you have a history of allergies, particularly to other antibiotics, it's crucial to let your healthcare provider know. This isn't just about Cephalexin; it's about keeping you safe. If someone has a known allergy to penicillin, for example, they should definitely communicate this to their doctor. It's similar to someone allergic to peanuts being cautious at a restaurant. A simple mention can prevent an allergic reaction and help ensure you receive a safe treatment plan.

Living with a pre-existing condition doesn't mean you have to avoid antibiotics altogether. It just means being proactive. Many people find success by keeping a health journal to track their symptoms and medications. This can help you notice patterns and communicate better with your healthcare provider. You might jot down when you take Cephalexin, how you're feeling, and any changes in your condition. This information can be incredibly valuable in guiding your treatment.

In summary, managing pre-existing conditions while taking Cephalexin requires awareness and communication. Don't hesitate to ask questions and share your health history with your healthcare provider. You want to ensure that all your health pieces fit together harmoniously, leading to a successful recovery. With the right approach and support, you can navigate your treatment with confidence, knowing you're taking the best steps for your overall health.

CHAPTER 6

Cephalexin for Specific Infections

When it comes to treating specific infections, Cephalexin can be a valuable tool in your healthcare toolkit. You might wonder, "What kind of infections is this medication used for?" or "How does it work for different conditions?" Let's dive into these questions and explore how Cephalexin can help manage various infections.

First off, think of Cephalexin as a dependable friend in the fight against bacterial infections. It belongs to a class of antibiotics known as cephalosporins, which are often used to treat a range of infections. Many people are familiar with it when it comes to treating skin infections, such as those pesky boils or cellulitis. Picture this: you're at a summer barbecue, and someone accidentally scrapes their arm on a rusty fence. A few days later, the scrape looks red and swollen. That's where Cephalexin can come into play. It helps fight the bacteria that might be causing the infection, allowing the wound to heal properly.

Now, let's not forget about ear infections, especially in children. They're as common as a rainy day. If a child has a painful ear infection, you might see them tugging at their ear and crying for comfort. Parents often worry about how to ease their child's discomfort and get them back to their playful selves. In these cases, doctors may prescribe Cephalexin to help clear the infection, giving parents peace of mind and kids a chance to play without pain.

But it's not just about children. Cephalexin is also effective for urinary tract infections (UTIs), which can affect anyone, regardless of age. Many people experience the discomfort of a UTI, characterized by a burning sensation when urinating and frequent bathroom trips. It can feel frustrating and disruptive to daily life. Cephalexin can help alleviate these symptoms by targeting the bacteria responsible for the infection, allowing you to return to your routine without constant worry. You might also encounter Cephalexin in treating respiratory infections, such as pneumonia. Picture an elderly relative who develops a persistent cough, along with fever and shortness of breath. These symptoms could indicate a respiratory infection. Doctors might prescribe Cephalexin to help tackle the bacteria causing the problem. By addressing the infection early, you can potentially prevent more serious complications.

But what happens if you have a pre-existing condition while dealing with one of these infections? Many people with conditions like asthma or diabetes worry about how antibiotics might affect their health. The good news is that Cephalexin is generally well-tolerated, but it's always wise to have an open conversation with your healthcare provider. They can help assess any potential interactions and tailor the treatment to your specific needs.

You might find it helpful to keep a record of how your body responds to Cephalexin if you have a chronic condition. For example, if you notice that your asthma seems to worsen after starting the antibiotic, this information is crucial for your doctor to know.

It's like being your own health detective—collecting clues that can lead to a better understanding of how different treatments affect you. As you can see, Cephalexin plays a significant role in managing various infections, from skin and ear infections to UTIs and respiratory issues. By recognizing the potential of this antibiotic, you can take proactive steps to address infections effectively. Remember, you're not alone in this journey. Your healthcare provider is there to guide you, ensuring that you receive the best care tailored to your unique health situation.

So, the next time you or a loved one faces an infection, consider how Cephalexin might fit into the picture. With the right approach and support, you can tackle these infections head-on, allowing you to focus on what really matters—getting back to your life, pain-free and healthy.

6.1 Skin Infections and Wound Care

When it comes to skin infections and wound care, understanding the role of medications like Cephalexin can make a world of difference in recovery. You might be wondering, "What kind of skin infections does this medication help with?" or "How can I take care of a wound properly?" Let's explore these questions in a way that makes sense and feels relatable.

Imagine it's a sunny afternoon, and your child is playing outside, climbing trees and racing bikes. But then, a tumble leads to a scraped knee. At first, it seems like just a minor injury, but a few days later, you notice redness and swelling around the wound. This is where a skin infection might be starting, and Cephalexin could be part of the solution. This antibiotic works by fighting off bacteria, helping the body heal while keeping the infection from getting worse.

But skin infections aren't just for kids. Adults can face them too, whether it's from a small cut or a more significant wound, like after surgery. You might have a friend who recently had a procedure and is worried about keeping their incision clean and free from infection. The doctor might prescribe Cephalexin to help ensure that the healing process goes smoothly.

Now, when it comes to wound care, you may wonder what steps to take. Proper wound care is crucial in preventing infections. It's a bit like gardening—if you want a beautiful flower to bloom, you must nurture the soil. Similarly, to help a wound heal, you need to keep it clean and protected. Start by washing your hands thoroughly before touching the wound. This simple act can help prevent harmful bacteria from entering.

After cleaning the wound gently with soap and water, you can apply an over-the-counter antibiotic ointment if recommended. Cover it with a clean bandage to protect it from dirt and bacteria. You might be surprised at how many people overlook this step, thinking that air exposure is best. While it's true that fresh air is essential, keeping the wound covered can actually help it heal faster and prevent infection.

If you notice signs of infection, such as increased redness, warmth, or drainage, it's essential to reach out to your healthcare provider. Many people hesitate to seek help, thinking it's just part of the healing process, but prompt attention can make a big difference. For instance, a neighbor might have ignored the initial signs of infection, thinking it would resolve on its own, only to find themselves facing a more severe issue weeks later. Now, let's talk about pre-existing conditions and how they play a role in managing skin infections. Many individuals have conditions like diabetes, which can complicate wound healing. If you or someone you know has diabetes, you might worry about how a simple scrape could lead to significant complications. In such cases, healthcare providers often take extra precautions. They might recommend more frequent monitoring of the wound and a closer look at any signs of infection.

You might be interested to know that the key to managing these risks often lies in education. For example, understanding the importance of keeping blood sugar levels stable can significantly impact healing. It's about being proactive—just like you would check the oil in your car to keep it running smoothly.

In summary, when it comes to skin infections and wound care, Cephalexin can be a valuable ally. By understanding how to care for wounds properly and recognizing when to seek medical help, you can take control of your healing journey. Whether it's a child's scraped knee or an adult's surgical wound, proper care makes all the difference. Remember, staying informed and proactive can help you and your loved ones enjoy healthy, infection-free skin.

6.2 Urinary Tract Infections (UTIs)

Urinary tract infections, or UTIs, are a common health concern that can affect people of all ages, but women, in particular, seem to have a knack for experiencing them. If you've ever had a UTI, you know it can feel like a relentless discomfort, almost like your bladder is protesting against the world. You might wonder, "What causes these pesky infections, and how can I get rid of them quickly?"

Let's dive into the world of UTIs, where personal experiences and practical advice can help shed light on this often frustrating issue. Picture this: it's the end of a long day, and you finally settle down for some well-deserved relaxation. Suddenly, you feel that familiar urge to run to the bathroom. But this time, something feels off. You find yourself making multiple trips, and each time, it's less than satisfying. This scenario is all too familiar for many people.

UTIs usually occur when bacteria enter the urinary tract and begin to multiply. This could happen after a long hike in the woods or simply due to dehydration. Many people might be surprised to learn that a lack of water intake can make them more susceptible to infections. Staying hydrated helps flush out bacteria, making it an essential part of prevention.

When it comes to treatment, antibiotics like Cephalexin can often step in to save the day. It's like having a trusty sidekick during a superhero battle—effective and ready to fight off the invading bacteria. However, you might wonder if there are other steps you can take to relieve your symptoms while waiting for the antibiotics to kick in. First, many people swear by drinking plenty of water. It's almost like nature's remedy. You might also hear that cranberry juice can help, although the science is mixed on this. Still, sipping on a glass may bring you some comfort, especially when you're trying to flush out your system.

Some individuals have personal stories of how they learned to manage UTIs effectively. A friend of mine shared her experience of suffering from recurrent UTIs. After countless trips to the doctor, she realized that certain habits were making her more prone to these infections. She started drinking more water, learned to wipe correctly after using the bathroom, and made it a point to urinate after intimate moments. These little changes made a world of difference in her life.

For many people, the symptoms of a UTI can range from mild to severe. You might experience burning during urination, a persistent urge to go, and sometimes even back pain. If you notice blood in your urine or have a fever, it's crucial to contact your healthcare provider. Many individuals worry that they're overreacting, but it's better to be safe than sorry. Ignoring symptoms could lead to complications or a longer recovery time.

It's also essential to recognize that some people may have pre-existing conditions that complicate UTIs. For instance, older adults may have other health issues that can make it harder to manage infections.

If you have a loved one in this category, consider being proactive by encouraging them to stay hydrated and seek medical advice if they notice any signs of discomfort.

Urinary tract infections can be a nuisance, but with the right knowledge and proactive steps, you can tackle them head-on. Whether it's through drinking more water, using antibiotics like Cephalexin, or simply being aware of your body's signals, managing UTIs is all about taking charge. So, if you find yourself in a bathroom scramble, remember that you're not alone in this experience. With a little care and attention, you can keep those pesky infections at bay and enjoy your daily life without constant interruptions.

6.3 Respiratory Infections (Sinusitis, Bronchitis)

When we think about respiratory infections, two common culprits often come to mind: sinusitis and bronchitis. Both can make you feel miserable, and if you've ever dealt with either of them, you probably remember that distinct feeling of congestion and discomfort. You might wonder what exactly causes these infections and how they differ from one another. Let's unpack this together in a way that feels relatable and easy to digest. Imagine waking up one morning, ready to take on the day. But as you get out of bed, you feel a heavy pressure in your forehead. You try to shake it off, thinking it might just be a result of a bad night's sleep. But as the day goes on, the pressure intensifies, and soon you find yourself sneezing, sniffling, and feeling downright fatigued. This scenario might sound familiar, and it could very well be sinusitis at play.

Sinusitis, often referred to as a sinus infection, occurs when the sinuses (the air-filled spaces in your skull) become inflamed. This inflammation can stem from allergies, a cold, or even environmental irritants. When the sinuses get blocked, mucus can build up, leading to that frustrating pressure and discomfort. Many people worry about the symptoms lasting too long, which can sometimes lead them to seek medical help.

Now, let's talk about bronchitis. You might recall a time when a persistent cough kept you awake at night, making you wonder if you were coming down with something serious. Bronchitis happens when the bronchial tubes (the airways that lead to your lungs) become inflamed, often due to a viral infection.

You might feel a tightness in your chest, and that annoying cough may produce mucus. This situation can feel like a never-ending cycle of discomfort. So, how do we address these pesky infections? Many people turn to antibiotics like Cephalexin, especially if there's a bacterial component involved. However, you might be surprised to learn that most sinus infections are viral in nature, which means antibiotics won't help much. Instead, a warm compress on your face, plenty of fluids, and over-the-counter decongestants might provide some relief.

A good friend of mine often gets sinus infections during allergy season. After a few rounds of antibiotics, she realized that managing her allergies proactively helped minimize her sinus issues. She started using saline nasal sprays and even invested in an air purifier. Those little changes made a world of difference for her.

When it comes to bronchitis, the approach can vary depending on whether it's acute or chronic. Acute bronchitis often clears up on its own, but chronic bronchitis requires more attention, especially for those with underlying health conditions like asthma. You might wonder about the role of smoking in this. Smokers are at a higher risk for chronic bronchitis, and quitting can significantly improve their lung health.

It's also essential to listen to your body. If you've been coughing for more than three weeks, or if you're experiencing shortness of breath or a fever, it's time to reach out to your healthcare provider. Many people worry about whether their symptoms are severe enough to warrant a visit, but better to check in than to risk complications down the road.

Respiratory infections like sinusitis and bronchitis can feel overwhelming, but with the right information and care, you can manage them effectively. Whether it's using medications like Cephalexin, exploring home remedies, or making lifestyle changes, there are plenty of ways to tackle these infections head-on. So, the next time you feel that familiar pressure in your sinuses or that nagging cough, remember that you have the tools to combat it. You're not alone in this; many people share these experiences, and together, we can navigate the ups and downs of respiratory health.

CHAPTER 7

Cephalexin vs. Other Antibiotics

When it comes to treating infections, there are a lot of antibiotics to choose from, and it can feel a bit overwhelming. In this chapter, we're diving into the world of Cephalexin and how it stacks up against other antibiotics. You might wonder why one antibiotic is prescribed over another, and it all boils down to the type of infection you're dealing with and how your body reacts to different medications.

Imagine your child has come down with an ear infection, which is all too common. You might recall a trip to the doctor where they prescribe amoxicillin. It's a go-to antibiotic for many pediatric infections. But what if you were prescribed Cephalexin instead? You'd probably want to know why. Cephalexin belongs to a class of antibiotics called cephalosporins, while amoxicillin is part of the penicillin family. Both are effective but work in slightly different ways. Cephalexin is often used for skin infections, respiratory infections, and urinary tract infections. It's like having a toolbox full of different tools, each designed for a specific job.

Let's look at a real-life scenario. A few months ago, my neighbor, a retired teacher, found himself with a painful skin infection. After a quick visit to the clinic, he was given Cephalexin. I remember him saying, "I didn't even know there were different antibiotics for skin infections!" This just goes to show how many people are in the dark about these medications.

You might be curious about how Cephalexin compares to other antibiotics like ciprofloxacin, which is often used for more serious infections, including certain types of bacterial diarrhea and respiratory infections. While both can be effective, they work best against different bacteria. Ciprofloxacin is a fluoroquinolone and is often reserved for more complicated cases due to its potency. Then there's doxycycline, another common antibiotic that's often prescribed for respiratory infections and acne. It's a member of the tetracycline family and can be effective against a broader range of bacteria. You might hear a friend say they were prescribed doxycycline for a nasty case of acne, and that's because it works well for that purpose.

Many people worry about antibiotic resistance, which has become a hot topic in recent years. This is when bacteria adapt and become resistant to medications, making infections harder to treat. Using the right antibiotic at the right time is crucial. That's why doctors carefully consider your specific infection when prescribing. For example, if someone has a simple urinary tract infection, a doctor might start with Cephalexin. But if the infection is more complex, they might opt for a different antibiotic to ensure they're targeting the right bacteria. It's kind of like choosing the right route on a road trip—you want to pick the path that gets you to your destination the fastest and most efficiently.

As we compare these antibiotics, it's essential to consider side effects too. While Cephalexin is generally well-tolerated, some people experience stomach upset or allergic reactions. You might remember a friend who had to switch antibiotics because of side effects, which is not uncommon.

So, in the battle of Cephalexin versus other antibiotics, there isn't a one-size-fits-all answer. It all comes down to the specific type of infection, the bacteria involved, and individual patient factors. Next time you or a loved one needs an antibiotic, remember that understanding the differences can help ease some of that anxiety. You're not just choosing a medication; you're participating in a careful decision-making process that prioritizes your health.

7.1 How It Compares to Other Common Antibiotics

When it comes to treating infections, antibiotics are often our first line of defense. You might wonder how Cephalexin stacks up against other common antibiotics like amoxicillin, doxycycline, and azithromycin. Understanding these differences can help you appreciate why your doctor might choose one over the others.

Let's start with amoxicillin, a familiar name in the antibiotic world. You've probably heard about it, especially when it comes to kids' ear infections or strep throat. It's part of the penicillin family and works wonders against certain bacteria. For many common infections, amoxicillin is often the go-to choice due to its effectiveness and relatively mild side effects. However, if a child doesn't respond to amoxicillin, a doctor might switch to Cephalexin.

Cephalexin is a member of the cephalosporin family, which means it has a slightly broader spectrum of action. It's especially good for skin infections, respiratory tract infections, and urinary tract infections. Picture it as a multi-tool: versatile enough to tackle various tasks. A friend of mine recently had a stubborn skin infection that didn't budge with amoxicillin. When she switched to Cephalexin, she noticed improvement within just a couple of days. It was a great reminder that sometimes a different approach can make all the difference.

Now, let's talk about doxycycline, which you might hear about when discussing more severe infections or even acne. Doxycycline is a tetracycline antibiotic and is effective against a wide range of bacteria. You might know someone who had to take doxycycline for a bad respiratory infection. While it can tackle serious issues, it also comes with some caveats. For example, it's not suitable for young children or pregnant women due to potential side effects on developing teeth and bones. So, when choosing between doxycycline and Cephalexin, a doctor will consider these factors.

Azithromycin, on the other hand, is often prescribed for respiratory infections like bronchitis or pneumonia. It's known for its convenience, as it typically requires fewer doses over a shorter period compared to other antibiotics. You might recall a friend telling you about how they felt better within a few days of starting azithromycin. That quick turnaround can be appealing, especially when you're feeling under the weather.

You might be wondering how these antibiotics compare in terms of side effects. Cephalexin is generally well-tolerated, but like any medication, it can cause issues. Some people might experience stomach upset or allergic reactions. You may have heard stories from friends or family who faced side effects from certain antibiotics, which can add to the stress of feeling sick.

Then there's the topic of antibiotic resistance, which has been making headlines lately. You may have noticed a growing awareness of how overusing antibiotics can lead to resistance, making infections harder to treat. This is why it's crucial to take antibiotics only when necessary and as prescribed. In this context, Cephalexin, along with other antibiotics, should be used thoughtfully to ensure they remain effective for future generations.

When comparing Cephalexin to other common antibiotics, it's clear that each one has its strengths and weaknesses. The choice often depends on the type of infection, the bacteria involved, and individual health considerations. Next time you or a loved one needs antibiotics, you'll have a better understanding of why your healthcare provider makes certain choices. It's all about finding the right tool for the job, ensuring that you get back on your feet as quickly and safely as possible.

7.2 When Cephalexin Is Preferred

When it comes to choosing the right antibiotic, you might wonder when Cephalexin is the best option. Understanding the specific situations where this medication shines can help you feel more informed and confident in discussions with your healthcare provider.

Let's start with a common scenario: skin infections. Imagine a busy parent who notices a painful, swollen area on their child's arm after a scrape from playing outside. This could be a sign of a bacterial skin infection, like cellulitis. In cases like these, Cephalexin often becomes the star of the show. Its effectiveness against certain bacteria that commonly cause skin infections makes it a preferred choice for doctors. My friend Sarah's son had a similar issue last summer. After a minor fall at the park, he developed a red, irritated patch on his knee. The pediatrician prescribed Cephalexin, and within a few days, his skin looked much better, allowing him to get back to his usual adventures.

Cephalexin is also handy for treating urinary tract infections (UTIs), especially in women. Picture this: you're at work, and suddenly, you start feeling an uncomfortable urgency to go to the bathroom. You might think it's just a bit of dehydration, but when that burning sensation hits, it's clear something's off. UTIs can be pesky, and when your doctor suspects a bacterial cause, Cephalexin is often the go-to antibiotic. Many women have experienced the relief of getting the right treatment quickly, allowing them to return to their daily routines without the discomfort that UTIs can cause.

Another area where Cephalexin shines is respiratory infections. While it might not be the first choice for viral infections like the common cold or flu, it can be effective against certain bacterial infections in the lungs, such as pneumonia or bronchitis. Let's say you've been battling a persistent cough and chest tightness. After seeing your doctor, they may decide that a bacterial infection is at play. In such cases, Cephalexin could be preferred, especially if they suspect specific bacteria that are responsive to it. One thing to keep in mind is that if you've had allergic reactions to penicillin, Cephalexin may also be a safer alternative. Many people worry about the potential for allergies when taking new medications. My aunt had a bad experience with amoxicillin years ago, so when she needed antibiotics for a tooth infection, her dentist opted for Cephalexin instead. This decision made her feel more comfortable knowing she was avoiding something that had caused her issues in the past.

You might also wonder about the role of Cephalexin in post-surgical care. After certain procedures, doctors may prescribe it to prevent infections, particularly in surgeries that involve the skin or soft tissues. Imagine a friend who just had surgery and is concerned about keeping the area clean and infection-free. By prescribing Cephalexin, the surgeon can help ensure that the healing process goes smoothly.

Cephalexin is preferred in various situations, particularly for skin infections, UTIs, certain respiratory infections, and as a preventive measure in post-surgical care. Knowing when this antibiotic is the right choice can help you better understand your treatment options and why your healthcare provider may recommend it. So, the next time you or someone you care about faces an infection, you'll have a clearer picture of why Cephalexin might be the right tool for the job.

CHAPTER 8

Consulting Your Healthcare Provider

When it comes to your health, one of the most important steps you can take is consulting your healthcare provider. You might wonder why this step is crucial, especially when dealing with infections that could require antibiotics like Cephalexin. Let's dive into this together.

Imagine you're feeling unwell and suspect you might have a bacterial infection. It's tempting to hop online and self-diagnose. But, as many people have discovered, the internet can be a double-edged sword. You might read about symptoms that match yours and become convinced you need an antibiotic. However, skipping the consultation can lead to problems. Without proper guidance, you may end up taking the wrong medication or even delaying appropriate treatment. For instance, let's think about Karen, a busy mother of two. One day, she started experiencing severe pain and swelling in her foot. After a quick search online, she thought she had an infection and asked her husband to pick up some antibiotics from the pharmacy. But when she finally visited her doctor, it turned out to be a sprained ankle—not an infection at all. If she had consulted her healthcare provider first, she could have avoided unnecessary worry and medication.

Now, you might be wondering what exactly you should discuss during your appointment. Start with your symptoms. Be honest and detailed. For example, if you've had a cough that just won't quit or a painful skin rash, sharing how long you've been feeling this way is vital. Your doctor will appreciate the information, and it will help them make an informed decision about your treatment options.

Don't be shy about asking questions, either! Many people worry about seeming bothersome when they ask about side effects or the necessity of a specific medication. But your health is your priority, and it's completely reasonable to seek clarity. If your doctor prescribes Cephalexin, you might ask how it works, what side effects to look out for, or how it differs from other antibiotics. This way, you'll not only be informed but also feel more in control of your treatment journey.

Another important aspect of consulting your healthcare provider is discussing any pre-existing conditions you may have. Let's say you've been living with diabetes for years. It's essential to inform your doctor about your condition, as it can affect how your body responds to medications. For example, if you get prescribed Cephalexin for a UTI, your doctor might monitor your blood sugar levels more closely, ensuring everything stays balanced.

After you leave your appointment, don't forget to follow up! If your doctor recommended a specific dosage or treatment plan, sticking to it is essential. If you notice any unusual symptoms after starting a new medication, like Cephalexin, reach out to your provider. Many people underestimate the importance of this step, thinking it's unnecessary to call for what might seem like minor side effects. But remember, early communication can often prevent larger issues down the line.

Consulting your healthcare provider is a key step in managing your health effectively. From accurately diagnosing your condition to tailoring a treatment plan that fits your needs, a good provider-patient relationship can make all the difference. By being proactive, asking questions, and keeping the lines of communication open, you'll empower yourself to navigate your health journey with confidence. So, the next time something feels off, don't hesitate to reach out. Your health is worth it!

8.1 Questions to Ask Before Taking Cephalexin

When your doctor prescribes Cephalexin, you might find yourself with a mix of curiosity and concern. After all, taking any medication is a big step, and it's essential to feel informed and confident about your choice. So, what should you ask before diving into this treatment? Let's explore some key questions that can help you understand what you're getting into. You might wonder, "What exactly is Cephalexin, and how does it work?" This is a great starting point. Cephalexin is an antibiotic that helps your body fight off certain types of bacterial infections. It's commonly used for skin infections, respiratory infections, and urinary tract infections. Understanding how it works can help ease your mind. Knowing that it targets bacteria rather than viruses can clarify why it's prescribed for specific issues but not for colds or the flu.

Next, consider asking about potential side effects. Many people worry about what might happen after taking a new medication. It's completely normal to feel anxious about this. Side effects can vary from mild stomach upset to more serious reactions. You might hear about nausea or diarrhea, which are not uncommon. By discussing these possibilities with your doctor, you can be prepared. Maybe they'll suggest tips to mitigate any discomfort, like taking medication with food.

Another important question is, "Are there any interactions with my current medications?" If you're taking other prescriptions or even over-the-counter supplements, it's crucial to know how they might interact with Cephalexin. For example, if you're on blood thinners, this could be particularly important to discuss. Your doctor can help you navigate any potential issues, ensuring your treatment plan is safe and effective.

You might also want to ask about the duration of treatment. Many people are eager to feel better, and it's helpful to know how long you'll be on Cephalexin. Your doctor can provide guidance on what to expect and when to follow up if your symptoms don't improve. For instance, if you're prescribed Cephalexin for a urinary tract infection, understanding that it's typically taken for seven to ten days can set your expectations. This can prevent the frustration of wondering when you'll start feeling better.

Another consideration is your medical history. You might ask, "Is there any reason I shouldn't take Cephalexin based on my past health issues?" If you have a history of allergies, particularly to penicillin or other cephalosporins, this is a crucial conversation to have. Your doctor will need this information to determine whether Cephalexin is a suitable choice for you.

You might also wonder about the importance of completing the full course of antibiotics. It's tempting to stop taking the medication once you start feeling better, but that can lead to issues like antibiotic resistance or a recurrence of the infection. Having a conversation about why it's vital to finish the entire prescription can help you understand the broader picture of antibiotic use.

Lastly, don't hesitate to ask, "What should I do if I miss a dose?" Life gets busy, and it's easy to forget. Your doctor can provide guidance on what to do if that happens—whether to take it as soon as you remember or wait until the next scheduled dose.

Asking the right questions before starting Cephalexin can empower you on your health journey. It's about creating a dialogue with your healthcare provider, ensuring you feel comfortable and informed about your treatment. Whether it's understanding the medication's effects or discussing your specific health needs, these conversations can help pave the way for a smoother recovery. So, the next time you're faced with a prescription, don't shy away from asking questions—your health is worth it!

8.2 Monitoring Progress and Follow-Up

When you're prescribed Cephalexin, you might feel a wave of relief, but it's just the beginning of your healing journey. Monitoring your progress and knowing when to follow up with your healthcare provider can make all the difference in your recovery. Let's dive into what this process looks like and why it's important.

First off, you might wonder what progress looks like. It's not always as clear-cut as checking a box. You may start to notice improvements, like less pain or fewer symptoms. For example, if you're treating a skin infection, you might see the redness and swelling gradually decrease. It's encouraging when you look in the mirror and see your skin returning to its normal tone. However, it's also normal to experience ups and downs during your treatment. That's why being mindful of your symptoms is crucial.

You might think, "How do I keep track of my progress?" One effective method is to maintain a simple journal. Jotting down daily notes about your symptoms, any side effects, and how you're feeling can provide valuable insight. For instance, if you notice that your stomach feels unsettled after taking the medication, writing it down can help your doctor make informed decisions during follow-up appointments. Plus, tracking your progress can give you a sense of control over your health journey.

Now, let's talk about follow-up appointments. Many people worry about whether they really need to return to the doctor. The answer is often yes! Regular follow-ups allow your healthcare provider to assess your response to Cephalexin. They'll want to know how you're feeling and if the antibiotic is effectively treating your infection. For instance, if you were prescribed Cephalexin for a urinary tract infection, your doctor might check in after a week to see if your symptoms have improved.

During these follow-ups, don't hesitate to share any concerns or side effects. You might say, "I'm feeling better, but I still have some discomfort," or "I've noticed some side effects." Your doctor is there to help you navigate these issues. They might adjust your dosage or suggest additional treatments based on what you share. It's all part of making sure you're on the right path to recovery. Another important aspect of monitoring your progress is understanding when to seek help sooner than planned. You might be thinking, "How do I know if something's wrong?" Pay attention to any new or worsening symptoms. If you notice a sudden spike in pain, fever, or any unusual reactions, it's vital to reach out to your healthcare provider right away. For example, if you're dealing with a skin infection and it suddenly gets redder or feels more painful, don't wait for your follow-up appointment—call your doctor.

Sometimes, despite taking Cephalexin, an infection can linger or not respond as expected. Many people worry about this scenario. It's essential to remember that every person's body reacts differently to medications. If you're still feeling unwell after completing your course, don't hesitate to discuss this with your healthcare provider. They may recommend further tests or a different treatment plan to get you back on track.

In summary, monitoring your progress while taking Cephalexin is about staying engaged in your own healthcare. It's about tracking your symptoms, keeping an open line of communication with your doctor, and knowing when to seek help. By actively participating in your recovery, you can better understand your body and make informed decisions that lead to healing. Remember, you're not alone on this journey; your healthcare provider is there to support you every step of the way.

8.3 What to Do If Symptoms Persist

When you're taking Cephalexin, you likely expect to feel better within a few days. However, sometimes the symptoms just don't seem to fade. You might wonder, "What should I do if my symptoms persist?" It's a common concern, and addressing it promptly can make a big difference in your recovery.

First things first: don't panic. It's not unusual for some infections to take longer to clear up, but it's crucial to listen to your body. Imagine this scenario: Sarah, a busy mom, was prescribed Cephalexin for a stubborn urinary tract infection. After a week, she noticed that while her symptoms had improved a little, she still felt discomfort. Instead of waiting and hoping it would go away, she reached out to her healthcare provider. This proactive approach helped her get the right treatment sooner rather than later. If you find yourself in a similar situation, here's a straightforward action plan. Start by making a list of your symptoms. Be specific. Instead of saying "I feel bad," try "I still have burning when I urinate, and my lower back hurts." This detailed information can be incredibly helpful for your doctor in determining the next steps.

Next, reach out to your healthcare provider. Many people worry about being a nuisance or think their concerns aren't serious enough. But remember, your doctor is there to help you. You might say, "I've been taking the medication as prescribed, but I'm still experiencing symptoms." This kind of honest communication is vital. Your doctor might recommend further tests, a different antibiotic, or additional treatments based on your feedback.

Another important aspect to consider is whether you have any underlying conditions that might be affecting your recovery. For example, if you have a history of recurrent urinary tract infections, it could mean that Cephalexin isn't the right choice this time.

Engaging in an open dialogue with your doctor about your medical history can provide context for your symptoms. Many people wonder about the timeline for improvement. It's understandable to feel frustrated if you expected to be well by now. You might find it helpful to think about the body's healing process as a marathon, not a sprint. Some infections require more time and attention than others. If you're still not feeling better after completing your course of Cephalexin, don't hesitate to check back in with your healthcare provider for guidance.

In addition to following up with your doctor, consider some self-care strategies. Staying hydrated is essential, especially for urinary tract infections. Drinking plenty of water can help flush out bacteria and support your healing process. You might also find relief with heat therapy; a warm compress on your abdomen can help ease discomfort. These small steps can complement your treatment and provide you with some comfort during a challenging time.

Lastly, keep in mind that persistence doesn't mean something is wrong with you. Everyone's body reacts differently to medications, and it's perfectly okay to seek further assistance. If your symptoms continue despite following the prescribed treatment, you deserve to understand why and explore other options.

If your symptoms persist while taking Cephalexin, the key is to stay engaged with your healthcare provider and advocate for yourself. Take note of your symptoms, reach out for help, and don't hesitate to explore alternative treatments if necessary. Your health journey is important, and taking these proactive steps can lead you toward feeling better sooner. Remember, you're not alone; many have walked this path, and reaching out for help is a sign of strength, not weakness.

CHAPTER 9

Lifestyle Tips During Antibiotic Treatment

When you're on antibiotics, it can feel like a whirlwind of medical terms and instructions. You might wonder how to take care of yourself during this time and what lifestyle changes can help you feel better. The good news is that a few simple tweaks to your daily routine can make a significant difference in how you respond to treatment.

First, let's talk about hydration. Picture this: you're sipping a glass of water after taking your antibiotics, and you feel good about it. Staying hydrated is crucial when you're on antibiotics, especially if you're dealing with infections. Water helps flush out toxins and can ease some side effects. You might remember your friend Emma, who once struggled with an infection but felt better after committing to drink more water. She discovered that it not only helped with her recovery but also kept her energy levels up.

Another important aspect is nutrition. You might find that your appetite changes while taking antibiotics. Some people crave comfort food, while others might not feel like eating at all. Try to focus on a balanced diet filled with fruits, vegetables, whole grains, and lean proteins. Think of it as fueling your body's engine. When Sarah was on antibiotics for a sinus infection, she made it a point to include yogurt in her meals. The probiotics helped replenish her gut bacteria, which can get thrown off balance during antibiotic treatment. Plus, it tasted great with some fresh fruit!

You may also want to limit processed foods and sugars during this time. Processed foods can sometimes cause inflammation and make you feel sluggish. Instead, opt for whole foods that give you the vitamins and minerals your body needs to fight off infection. If you're unsure where to start, think about your favorite healthy meals and how you can incorporate them into your diet while on antibiotics. Don't forget about your gut health! You might have heard the term "gut microbiome" thrown around. It refers to the collection of bacteria in your digestive system, and antibiotics can disrupt this balance. Probiotics, found in foods like yogurt, sauerkraut, and kombucha, can help. If you're not a fan of those foods, consider talking to your healthcare provider about taking a probiotic supplement. It's a great way to support your gut while your body heals.

Rest is another vital part of the healing process. Many people worry about how much rest they should get. The truth is, your body does a lot of its healing while you sleep. If you find yourself feeling tired, don't hesitate to take that afternoon nap or go to bed a little earlier. Just think of it as your body's way of recharging its batteries. You might recall a time when you pushed through feeling unwell and paid for it later. Instead, give yourself permission to relax and take it easy when you need to.

Physical activity is important too, but you don't have to go overboard. Gentle exercise, like a leisurely walk or some light stretching, can boost your mood and energy. However, listen to your body. If you feel worn out, it's perfectly fine to take a break. For example, Mark decided to take short walks in his neighborhood while on antibiotics for a respiratory infection. He found it helped him feel more energized without overexerting himself.

Lastly, you might find that stress management becomes more crucial during your treatment. Stress can affect your immune system, so it's essential to find ways to relax. Whether it's through meditation, reading, or spending time with loved ones, carve out time for activities that bring you joy. Remember the last time you had a good laugh with friends? That kind of positive energy can do wonders for your well-being.

Managing your lifestyle while on antibiotics doesn't have to be complicated. Stay hydrated, focus on nutrition, prioritize rest, incorporate gentle exercise, and manage stress. Think of this time as an opportunity to nurture yourself and support your body in its healing journey. Many people have successfully navigated this path, and you can too!

Embrace these tips and give your body the care it needs to recover fully.

9.1 Importance of Hydration and Rest

When you're on antibiotics like cephalexin, you might hear a lot about hydration and rest. You might wonder why these two things are often stressed so much. After all, they seem simple enough. But in reality, they play a significant role in how well your body fights off infection and heals.

Let's start with hydration. Imagine your body as a well-tuned engine. Just like a car needs oil to run smoothly, your body needs water. When you're taking antibiotics, hydration helps your body flush out toxins and waste products. It can also help minimize some side effects that might pop up during treatment. Think back to the last time you were sick. Did you ever notice how a few extra glasses of water made you feel more energized?

For example, when my friend Jessica was on antibiotics for a severe sinus infection, she made it a point to drink at least eight glasses of water a day. She found that it helped her feel less fatigued and more alert. You might find yourself feeling sluggish when you're not drinking enough, and nobody likes that feeling when you're already unwell. Water can also help combat the dryness that some medications cause, making it easier to swallow and digest your food.

Now, let's talk about rest. When you're sick, your body goes into high gear to fight off the infection. This process can take a lot of energy. Just like your phone needs to be charged after a long day of use, your body needs rest to recover. You might have heard the old saying, "Sleep is the best medicine." It's true! Sleep helps your body repair itself and regenerate those important immune cells.

Take the story of my neighbor, who once battled a nasty bout of pneumonia. He was adamant about not taking time off work, thinking he could power through it. But he quickly learned that pushing himself only delayed his recovery. Once he decided to take a few days to rest, he noticed a significant improvement in how he felt. You might find that getting enough sleep helps you feel more like yourself again.

You might also wonder about the right balance between hydration and rest. It's important to remember that they go hand in hand. When you're well-hydrated, your body can function better, which can lead to more restful sleep. On the flip side, if you're not getting enough sleep, you might not feel thirsty or motivated to drink enough water. It's a bit of a cycle, and recognizing it can help you take charge of your health.

If you're unsure about how much water to drink or how to improve your sleep, start with small changes. Set reminders on your phone to take a drink of water every hour or try to establish a relaxing bedtime routine. This could include reading a book or practicing some gentle stretches. You might be surprised at how little changes can lead to significant improvements in your overall well-being.

Hydration and rest are essential when you're on antibiotics. They support your body in its fight against infection and help you bounce back more quickly. Think of them as your trusty sidekicks on the road to recovery. So, grab that water bottle, find a cozy spot, and give your body the care it deserves. You'll be glad you did!

9.2 Foods That Support Recovery

When you're on antibiotics like cephalexin, it's not just about taking the right medication; what you eat plays a crucial role in your recovery, too. You might wonder, "What foods can really help me heal?" Let's explore some options that can support your body as it fights off infection. First off, think about your immune system as a defense team. Just like a sports team needs the right players to succeed, your body needs certain nutrients to keep your immune system strong. Foods rich in vitamins and minerals can give that team a serious boost.

One of the star players in this recovery game is yogurt. You might have heard about probiotics—the good bacteria that help keep your gut healthy. When you take antibiotics, they can disrupt the balance of these bacteria, leading to digestive issues. Eating yogurt can help replenish those good bacteria. I remember when my cousin took antibiotics for a bad infection. She started adding yogurt to her breakfast every morning, and it really helped her stomach feel better. Next, let's talk about fruits and vegetables. These colorful foods are packed with vitamins and antioxidants that help your body recover. For instance, vitamin C is well-known for its immune-boosting properties, and you can find it in oranges, strawberries, and bell peppers. You might even recall your grandmother insisting you eat your veggies whenever you were sick; she knew what she was talking about!

Incorporating leafy greens like spinach and kale into your meals is another great idea. They're rich in vitamins A and C and can help with overall health. Try tossing them into a smoothie or making a refreshing salad. I often whip up a green smoothie when I'm not feeling my best—it's a simple way to get a nutrient-packed boost without too much effort.

Don't forget about lean proteins, either. Foods like chicken, fish, and legumes are essential for rebuilding tissues and supporting recovery. If you enjoy cooking, a comforting chicken soup can be both nourishing and soothing when you're under the weather. A friend of mine swears by her mom's homemade chicken soup whenever she feels sick. It's like a warm hug in a bowl! Healthy fats, like those found in avocados, nuts, and olive oil, are also important. They help reduce inflammation and can provide lasting energy, which is especially useful when your body is working hard to heal. You might try adding slices of avocado to your toast or snacking on a handful of almonds throughout the day.

Lastly, hydration is crucial, and while water is always the best choice, herbal teas can be a soothing option as well. Peppermint tea can aid digestion, while ginger tea may help reduce nausea. You might find yourself wrapped up in a cozy blanket with a cup of tea, feeling comforted as you take care of your body.

So, as you navigate your antibiotic treatment, think about the foods that can support your recovery. You don't need to make drastic changes—just incorporating a few nutrient-rich foods into your diet can make a big difference. Listen to your body and give it what it needs to get back on track. With a little care in the kitchen, you'll be fueling your recovery and feeling better before you know it!

9.3 Managing Digestive Side Effects

Taking antibiotics can feel like a double-edged sword. On one hand, they're fighting off that nasty infection, but on the other, they can cause some digestive side effects that leave you feeling uncomfortable. You might wonder, "What can I do to manage these issues?" Let's dive into some practical strategies to help you navigate this tricky situation.

First, let's talk about one of the most common side effects: an upset stomach. Many people experience nausea, diarrhea, or bloating when they start a course of antibiotics. It can feel like your stomach is in turmoil, but there are ways to ease that discomfort. One helpful tip is to take your antibiotics with food. You might be surprised by how much of a difference this can make! Having a small meal or snack can create a buffer in your stomach, making the medication easier to tolerate. Think about a simple bowl of oatmeal or some toast—something easy on the stomach that can help settle things down.

Another thing to consider is hydration. When your stomach isn't happy, it's essential to drink plenty of water. Staying hydrated helps your body flush out toxins and can prevent dehydration, especially if you're experiencing diarrhea. You might even find sipping on ginger tea soothing. I remember a friend who had a rough time with antibiotics. She discovered ginger tea was a game-changer for her nausea, and now she swears by it whenever she feels queasy.

Then, there's the issue of balancing out your gut flora. As we discussed earlier, antibiotics can disrupt the good bacteria in your gut. That's where probiotics come into play. You might have heard about them before; they're the good bacteria that can help restore balance in your digestive system. Yogurt, kefir, sauerkraut, and kimchi are all excellent sources. You might remember your grandmother eating fermented foods—she likely knew they were good for digestion!

If you're looking for something more convenient, many people turn to probiotic supplements. Just remember to check with your healthcare provider before starting any new supplements, especially while on antibiotics. They can help guide you on what's best for your specific situation.

Another effective strategy is to be mindful of what you eat. While it can be tempting to reach for comfort food, it might not always be the best choice. Spicy or fatty foods can further irritate your stomach. Instead, opt for bland, easily digestible foods like bananas, rice, applesauce, and toast—the classic "BRAT" diet. I've found that these foods not only help settle an upset stomach but can also be comforting during recovery.

Lastly, listen to your body. If you notice that certain foods trigger discomfort, it's okay to avoid them while you're on antibiotics. You might also want to keep a journal to track what you eat and how it makes you feel. This way, you can identify patterns and find out what works best for you.

Remember, managing digestive side effects is all about finding what helps you feel better. With a little care and attention to your diet, you can support your digestive health while your antibiotics do their job. You're not alone in this; many people face similar challenges, and with some simple strategies, you can ease those uncomfortable side effects and focus on feeling better.

CHAPTER 10

Dealing with Missed or Incorrect Doses

When you're on antibiotics, sticking to your dosing schedule is crucial. But life happens, right? Maybe you forgot to take a dose, or perhaps you accidentally took too much. You might be wondering, "What should I do now?" Let's break it down and make this topic a bit easier to navigate.

First off, if you miss a dose, don't panic. It happens to everyone at some point. The key is to act quickly. Most of the time, you can take the missed dose as soon as you remember, but there are a few caveats. For instance, if it's almost time for your next dose, just skip the missed one. Don't double up! This could lead to an overdose, which might cause more problems than it solves.

Imagine this: you're in the middle of your workday, and your mind is racing with tasks. You meant to take your antibiotic with breakfast but completely forgot. When you finally remember, you check the clock and see it's nearly time for lunch. In this case, just let it go and take your next dose on schedule. Trust me, it's better to stay safe than to risk upsetting your stomach or causing other side effects.

You might also be curious about what to do if you realize you've taken too much. If you suspect an overdose, it's essential to reach out to your healthcare provider or local poison control center immediately. They can guide you on the best steps to take based on how much you've taken and when. It's always better to err on the side of caution.

You might wonder how missing doses can impact your treatment. Well, antibiotics work best when taken consistently, so it's crucial to try to stay on track. Incomplete dosing can lead to your body not fully clearing the infection, which might cause it to come back or become resistant to the medication.

This is something you definitely want to avoid. To help you remember your doses, consider setting reminders on your phone or using a pill organizer. These simple tools can be lifesavers. I've heard stories from friends who struggled to remember their meds, but once they started using these methods, it made a world of difference. It's like having a little helper reminding you to take care of yourself!

You might also want to keep a medication log. It's a straightforward way to track what you've taken and when. This can be especially helpful if you have multiple medications or if you're taking antibiotics for a longer duration. Not only does it keep you organized, but it also provides valuable information for your healthcare provider if you need to discuss your treatment.

Finally, communication is key. If you're unsure about what to do after missing a dose or if you have concerns about the effectiveness of your treatment, don't hesitate to reach out to your healthcare provider. They're there to help and can provide the guidance you need. It's always better to ask questions and clarify things rather than stress about it alone.

Dealing with missed or incorrect doses can feel a bit overwhelming, but remember that it's a common issue. With some simple strategies and open communication with your healthcare provider, you can navigate these bumps in the road and stay on track with your treatment. Your health journey is important, and every step counts!

10.1 What to Do If You Miss a Dose

You're going about your day, and suddenly it hits you—you forgot to take your antibiotic dose. You might be feeling that little knot of anxiety in your stomach, thinking, "What now?" Don't worry; missing a dose is something most people experience at some point. Let's talk about what you should do if you find yourself in this situation.

First, take a deep breath. It's important to stay calm. If you remember your missed dose shortly after it was supposed to be taken, you can usually just take it as soon as you remember. For example, let's say you were supposed to take your antibiotic for breakfast, but you got busy with work and forgot. If it's still morning and you just realized it, go ahead and take it.

However, if it's almost time for your next dose, skip the missed one. Doubling up can lead to too much medication in your system, which can cause side effects or even make you feel worse. Think of it like trying to fill a glass of water. If the glass is already full, pouring in more will just make a mess.

You might wonder, "How do I prevent this from happening again?" One effective method is to set reminders on your phone. Many people find that a simple alarm or notification helps them remember their doses. I've heard stories from friends who use sticky notes on their fridge or bathroom mirror as visual reminders, which can be a fun and effective way to keep track.

It's also helpful to create a routine around taking your medication. If you take it at the same time as another daily activity—like brushing your teeth or having breakfast—it can make remembering easier. Imagine you're getting ready for bed, and you always take your antibiotic right after brushing your teeth. Over time, your brain will associate the two actions, making it less likely for you to forget.

If you realize you missed a dose and it's been several hours or even a day, don't panic. Just skip that dose and continue with your regular schedule. Most antibiotics can handle a missed dose without serious issues, but it's crucial to stay consistent moving forward.

Many people worry about what a missed dose could mean for their treatment. While it's best to take your medication as prescribed, missing one dose typically doesn't spell disaster. Just make sure to keep an eye on how you're feeling. If you start to notice that your symptoms are coming back or worsening, it's a good idea to reach out to your healthcare provider. They can help determine if you need to adjust your treatment plan. Also, don't forget to keep your healthcare provider in the loop. If you find yourself missing doses regularly, let them know. They might have suggestions or even consider adjusting your medication schedule to better fit your lifestyle.

If you miss a dose, just remember to stay calm. Take it as soon as you remember, unless it's almost time for your next dose, in which case, skip it. Use reminders and create routines to help you stay on track. And always feel free to reach out for advice if you're unsure about what to do. Your health is a journey, and sometimes, there are bumps along the way. But with a little organization and open communication, you can navigate these challenges like a pro!

10.2 Handling Overdoses Safely

Imagine this: You're feeling under the weather and taking your antibiotic as prescribed. You're on a mission to feel better, but in a moment of distraction—maybe a phone call or a busy day—you accidentally take more than the recommended dose. You might feel that sudden rush of panic. What should you do?

First, it's important to stay calm. Overdosing on antibiotics like amoxicillin is not something most people encounter often, but it can happen. The first thing you should do is figure out how much you took. Did you accidentally take an extra pill or two? Or did you go a little overboard? Knowing the details will help you understand your next steps.

If you realize you've taken more than prescribed, don't just sit there worrying. Call your healthcare provider or a poison control center right away. They are equipped to handle these situations and can provide you with the best advice based on your specific circumstances. You might wonder, "What can they do?" Well, they can assess your situation and let you know if you need to go to the hospital or if it's safe to stay at home and monitor your symptoms.

For example, I once heard a story about a friend who was feeling sick and mistakenly thought taking an extra dose would help her recover faster. She felt that wave of worry when she realized what she'd done. Thankfully, she called her doctor, who reassured her that, in her case, she just needed to drink plenty of water and keep an eye on how she felt. But not everyone is so lucky, which is why it's crucial to reach out for professional advice.

You might also wonder about the symptoms of an overdose. While most people don't experience severe side effects from taking too much amoxicillin, some might notice stomach upset, diarrhea, or a headache. If you find yourself feeling unwell, it's definitely a reason to seek medical attention. Think of your body as a finely tuned machine; too much of anything—even something beneficial like an antibiotic—can throw it off balance. One important thing to remember is to keep all medications out of reach, especially if you have little ones running around. Kids are naturally curious, and it's easy for them to grab something that looks like candy. Childproof containers and high shelves are great strategies to prevent accidental overdoses.

After the immediate situation is handled, it's a good time to reflect on how to avoid this in the future. Many people find it helpful to set a routine when taking medications. For example, if you take your antibiotics after a specific meal or while doing another daily activity—like brushing your teeth—this can make it easier to keep track of your doses and avoid confusion.

In the grand scheme of things, everyone makes mistakes from time to time. Handling an overdose safely is all about acting quickly and knowing who to contact. If you find yourself in a situation where you've taken too much medication, don't hesitate to reach out for help. Your health and safety come first, and there's always a way to navigate the bumps in the road. Remember, knowledge is power, and being informed can help you take control of your health journey.

10.3 Avoiding Antibiotic Resistance

Antibiotic resistance is a hot topic in medicine these days, and for good reason. You might have heard people talk about it, and you may be wondering why it matters so much to you, especially when you're trying to recover from an infection. Let's break it down. Imagine you've got a pesky ear infection. Your doctor prescribes amoxicillin, and you're hopeful it will kick that infection to the curb. But what happens if antibiotics are misused? Over time, the bacteria that cause infections can learn how to survive despite these medications. This is what we call antibiotic resistance. It's like a superhero bacteria that gets stronger every time it battles with antibiotics.

One of the most common ways resistance develops is when antibiotics are not taken as directed. For example, let's say you start feeling better after a few days on amoxicillin, and you decide to stop taking it. Many people think, "I feel fine, so why finish the whole bottle?" Well, this is a common mistake. By stopping too soon, you may leave behind a few bacteria that weren't completely wiped out. Those bacteria can adapt and become resistant.

There's a story I heard from a friend who had a similar experience. She was prescribed antibiotics for a urinary tract infection (UTI) and felt much better after just a few days. But instead of finishing the entire course, she stopped taking them. A few weeks later, the infection came back, but this time, the antibiotics didn't work as well. She ended up in a frustrating cycle of trying different medications, many of which were less effective.

You might wonder what else contributes to antibiotic resistance. Overprescribing antibiotics is a big factor. Sometimes, people go to the doctor expecting a prescription for antibiotics, even when they have a viral infection like the flu or a cold. These infections won't respond to antibiotics, but that pressure can lead to unnecessary prescriptions.

Another culprit? Sharing antibiotics. You might think it's harmless to lend a friend some leftover pills from a past infection. However, this can lead to taking the wrong medication for their illness, which can cause resistance to develop in the bacteria they have. It's essential to only take antibiotics prescribed specifically for you, for the infection you have.

So, how can you help avoid antibiotic resistance? Here are some practical tips:

1. **Follow the Instructions**: Always take your antibiotics exactly as your doctor prescribes. Finish the entire course, even if you start feeling better.
2. **Don't Pressure Your Doctor**: If you visit a healthcare provider and they tell you antibiotics aren't necessary, trust their expertise. It's okay to ask questions, but also be open to alternative treatments.
3. **Never Share Medications**: Keep your antibiotics to yourself. What works for you may not be suitable for someone else's illness.
4. **Practice Good Hygiene**: Simple habits like washing your hands frequently can help

prevent infections, reducing the need for antibiotics in the first place.
5. **Stay Informed**: You might wonder how you can stay educated on this topic. Ask your healthcare provider for resources or check reputable websites for information about antibiotics and their proper use.

By taking these steps, you're not just looking out for yourself; you're helping to protect your community. Every time you use antibiotics responsibly, you contribute to a larger fight against antibiotic resistance. It's a team effort, and you play a vital role. The next time you find yourself reaching for those antibiotics, remember: you're part of a bigger picture that can help ensure these life-saving medications work effectively for everyone.

CHAPTER 11

Myths and Misconceptions About Antibiotics

When it comes to antibiotics, myths and misconceptions abound, and they can lead to confusion, misuse, and ultimately, health risks. Let's explore some of the most common myths surrounding antibiotics, debunk them, and clarify the truth so you can make informed decisions about your health.

One of the most prevalent myths is that antibiotics can treat any infection. You might have heard someone say, "I have a cold; I need antibiotics!" But here's the reality: antibiotics are designed to fight bacterial infections, not viral ones. So, if you catch a cold or the flu, antibiotics won't help you recover. It's like trying to use a hammer to screw in a nail—you're using the wrong tool for the job. Many people don't realize that a cold, caused by a virus, will run its course naturally, while a bacterial infection, like strep throat, does need antibiotics.

There's also a misconception that if you feel better after just a few days of taking antibiotics, you can stop the medication. This is a common situation many face. For example, imagine a parent whose child is prescribed amoxicillin for an ear infection. After three days, the child seems to be back to their usual playful self. The parent might think, "Great! They're better!" However, stopping the antibiotics early can leave some bacteria alive, allowing them to multiply and potentially cause a relapse or more severe infection. It's crucial to follow the full course as directed, even if you or your child feel better before finishing it.

Another myth is that antibiotics are safe to take whenever you feel sick. Many people worry about becoming dependent on antibiotics or suffering side effects, leading them to take them whenever they think they might be ill. But here's the truth: every time you use antibiotics unnecessarily, you're increasing your risk of antibiotic resistance, which makes these vital medications less effective in the future. Think of it like borrowing your neighbor's lawn mower. If you borrow it too often, they might not want to lend it to you the next time you actually need it.

You might also wonder if it's okay to share antibiotics with friends or family. "They've had the same symptoms I had; surely this will help them too!" Unfortunately, this is another dangerous myth. Just because you were prescribed antibiotics for a certain infection doesn't mean they are appropriate for someone else. Different infections require different treatments, and sharing can lead to ineffective treatment or harmful side effects. Imagine if someone gave you a friend's leftover allergy medication that they were allergic to—yikes!

There's a belief that antibiotics can cure everything, from a simple headache to a sprained ankle. This myth can stem from a desire to find a quick fix for any ailment. While antibiotics are crucial for treating bacterial infections, they do not address everything. Sometimes, the best approach is rest, hydration, and time. For instance, many people seek antibiotics for digestive issues, thinking they'll help. However, digestive problems often stem from dietary choices or infections that don't require antibiotics.

Lastly, many people think that all antibiotics work the same way or are interchangeable. For example, you might have heard someone say, "I took penicillin last year; this time, I'll just grab some amoxicillin." While they are related, these antibiotics are not identical. Just as not all tools are the same, not all antibiotics are effective against every bacterial infection. Using the wrong antibiotic can be ineffective or even harmful.

So, what can you do to combat these myths? Stay informed and ask questions. When your doctor prescribes antibiotics, don't hesitate to inquire about their purpose and how they work. Understanding why you need them can empower you to follow the treatment plan effectively. In the end, the key to managing antibiotics lies in understanding their role and using them responsibly. When we break down these misconceptions and rely on accurate information, we can protect our health and ensure antibiotics remain effective for those who truly need them. Knowledge is power, and with the right information, you can confidently navigate the world of antibiotics.

11.1 Understanding Antibiotic Resistance

Understanding antibiotic resistance is essential for anyone who has ever taken medication or cared for someone who has. You might wonder what antibiotic resistance really means and why it's such a big deal in today's world. Imagine this scenario: You're a parent who's just received a prescription for amoxicillin for your child's ear infection. You've heard that antibiotics are powerful tools in fighting infections. But what if I told you that over time, some bacteria can become resistant to these medications, making them less effective or even useless? This is what we mean by antibiotic resistance.

To break it down, antibiotics are designed to kill bacteria or inhibit their growth. However, not all bacteria are created equal. Some bacteria can survive exposure to antibiotics, and those that do are often referred to as "superbugs." Picture a video game where you're fighting a boss character. If you find a winning strategy, you might defeat that boss. But if the boss adapts and learns from your tactics, you could be in trouble. That's essentially how bacteria adapt and become resistant.

You might wonder how this happens. Well, it often starts with the overuse or misuse of antibiotics. Many people worry about taking medication for every sniffle or cough, thinking it's the quick fix to feeling better. But as we've discussed, antibiotics don't work against viral infections like the common cold or the flu. When antibiotics are prescribed unnecessarily, it gives bacteria a chance to learn how to resist them. It's like throwing a party and inviting all your friends, but not realizing that some of them were once in a rival gang. The more you expose bacteria to antibiotics, the greater the chance they will develop defenses against those drugs.

Let's consider a real-life example: an elderly person recovering from a urinary tract infection (UTI). If they've been treated with antibiotics multiple times over the years, the bacteria causing their infections may have become resistant. This can lead to longer hospital stays and more complicated treatments. It's like trying to fix a leaky faucet. If you keep using the same quick-fix solution, it might not work eventually, and you'll have to call in a plumber.

So why should you care about antibiotic resistance? Because it affects everyone. Imagine a world where common infections, like a simple strep throat or a post-surgical infection, could no longer be treated effectively. Hospitals could fill up with patients suffering from infections that don't respond to standard treatments. It's a scary thought, isn't it?

But there is hope! Understanding antibiotic resistance can help you play an active role in preventing it. You might be wondering, "What can I do?" Well, here are a few practical steps you can take:

- **Use antibiotics only when prescribed**: If your doctor suggests antibiotics, ask them why they're necessary. If it's a viral infection, it's better to focus on rest and hydration.

- **Follow the prescribed course**: If you start antibiotics, complete the entire course as directed, even if you feel better. It's like finishing a race—you want to cross the finish line, not stop halfway through.
- **Practice good hygiene**: Simple actions like washing your hands regularly and staying up to date on vaccinations can help prevent infections, reducing the need for antibiotics.
- **Educate others**: Share what you know about antibiotic resistance with friends and family. The more people are informed, the better we can work together to tackle this issue.

In summary, understanding antibiotic resistance is crucial for safeguarding our health and the effectiveness of these medications. By being informed and taking responsible actions, we can help ensure that antibiotics remain effective tools in our healthcare arsenal. Remember, it's not just about one prescription; it's about preserving the power of antibiotics for everyone in the future.

11.2 Are All Infections Treatable with Antibiotics?

You might be surprised to learn that not all infections are treatable with antibiotics. This is a common misconception, and it's important to understand why. Many people worry that antibiotics are a one-size-fits-all solution to every type of infection, but that's simply not the case.

Let's start with a simple analogy. Imagine your body as a bustling city, filled with all sorts of people, cars, and buildings. Some areas of the city are peaceful, while others might be in chaos. When a crisis hits, like a traffic jam or a broken water main, you need the right team to tackle the specific problem. In this analogy, antibiotics are like emergency responders, but they can only help with certain types of emergencies.

Antibiotics are effective against bacterial infections, such as strep throat or a urinary tract infection. When a doctor prescribes amoxicillin for your child's ear infection, it's because they suspect that bacteria are causing the problem. By targeting these bacteria, antibiotics can help the body heal faster and feel better. However, if your child has a cold or the flu—caused by viruses—antibiotics won't do a thing. It's like sending firefighters to deal with a flood; they just won't help in that situation.

You might wonder why it's so easy to confuse the two. After all, both bacterial and viral infections can have similar symptoms, like fever, fatigue, and cough. Many people mistakenly believe that if they're feeling unwell, a quick course of antibiotics will solve the problem. Unfortunately, taking antibiotics for viral infections not only won't help you feel better but can also contribute to antibiotic resistance. It's like overusing a tool until it breaks; the more you rely on antibiotics for conditions they can't treat, the less effective they become when you truly need them.

Let's consider a real-life scenario: you visit your doctor because you have a sore throat. After examining you, the doctor might say, "I think you have strep throat; let's test for it." If the test comes back positive, antibiotics like amoxicillin might be prescribed to help you recover. But if it turns out you have a viral infection instead, the doctor will likely recommend rest, hydration, and over-the-counter remedies to ease your symptoms. This highlights the importance of accurate diagnosis. It's essential for healthcare professionals to determine whether an infection is caused by bacteria or a virus before prescribing treatment. Sometimes, tests can be done to identify the culprit. Other times, it's a matter of the doctor's experience and knowledge.

Another key point to remember is that some infections are caused by fungi or parasites, neither of which can be treated with standard antibiotics. For instance, athlete's foot is a fungal infection that requires antifungal treatment, while malaria is a parasitic infection that needs specific medications. So, it's not just about distinguishing between bacterial and viral infections; understanding the type of infection is crucial for effective treatment.

You might find it helpful to consider preventative measures as well. Staying healthy can reduce the risk of infections altogether. Regular handwashing, keeping up with vaccinations, and maintaining a balanced diet are all important steps in keeping your immune system strong.

While antibiotics like amoxicillin are powerful tools for fighting bacterial infections, they are not a blanket solution for every illness. Understanding the differences between bacterial, viral, fungal, and parasitic infections can empower you to make informed decisions about your health. The next time you're feeling under the weather, remember to consult with your healthcare provider to find the best treatment for your specific situation. It's all about using the right tool for the right job—your health deserves nothing less!

11.3 Clearing Up Confusion About Side Effects

When it comes to taking antibiotics like amoxicillin, confusion about side effects is surprisingly common. You might have heard stories from friends or family about how they felt sick after taking their medication, leading you to wonder, "Is this normal? Should I be worried?" Let's take a closer look at what side effects really mean, why they happen, and how to approach them.

Imagine you've just been prescribed amoxicillin for your child's ear infection. You might feel a wave of relief, knowing that this antibiotic can help them feel better. But then you remember the stories you've heard about antibiotics causing stomach aches or rashes. You start to worry. You're not alone—many parents feel this way, and it's completely understandable.

So, what exactly are side effects? Simply put, they are unintended reactions to a medication. While we often think of side effects as negative, they can be a sign that the medication is working. For example, when amoxicillin is taken, it targets the bacteria causing the infection. In doing so, it can also affect some of the healthy bacteria in the gut, which might lead to mild gastrointestinal discomfort.

Now, let's say your child starts complaining of an upset stomach a few days into their treatment. This can be concerning, but it's important to remember that not everyone will experience side effects. Many people take amoxicillin without any issues. According to health experts, common side effects may include diarrhea, nausea, and mild rashes.

You might wonder how serious these side effects can be. For most people, they are mild and resolve on their own once the treatment is completed. Think of it as your body adjusting to the changes caused by the medication, much like how your taste buds adapt to a new flavor after a few bites. However, if the side effects become severe or your child shows signs of a more serious reaction, such as difficulty breathing or swelling of the face, that's when you should seek medical help immediately. It's essential to know the difference between mild discomfort and a serious reaction, which can often be accomplished with a simple phone call to your healthcare provider.

You might also be curious about how to minimize side effects. One practical tip is to take antibiotics with food, as this can help reduce stomach upset. Make sure your child is drinking plenty of fluids and eating a balanced diet to keep their system running smoothly. Sometimes, probiotics can also be beneficial, as they help restore the healthy bacteria in the gut that antibiotics can disrupt.

In another real-life scenario, imagine an elderly person being treated for a urinary tract infection with amoxicillin. They may have concerns about how it will affect their digestion, especially if they have a history of stomach issues. It's important for caregivers and loved ones to communicate openly about any changes in symptoms, whether positive or negative. Keeping a close eye on how they're feeling can help identify any problems early on.

Throughout this journey, open communication with healthcare professionals is crucial. If you have concerns about side effects, don't hesitate to ask questions. You might ask your doctor, "What side effects should I watch out for?" or "Are there alternatives that might have fewer side effects?" They can provide reassurance and guidance tailored to your specific situation.

While side effects can sound intimidating, they are often a normal part of the healing process when taking antibiotics like amoxicillin. By understanding what to expect and maintaining an open line of communication with healthcare providers, you can navigate this process with confidence. Remember, it's all about finding the right balance for your health and knowing when to reach out for help. Your well-being is worth it!

CHAPTER 12

Cephalexin in Special Populations

When it comes to taking medications like cephalexin, it's essential to consider how different groups of people might respond. From young children to the elderly and pregnant women, each group has unique needs and concerns. In this chapter, we'll explore how cephalexin fits into the lives of these special populations, ensuring that everyone gets the care they deserve.

Picture this: you're a parent whose child has developed a skin infection. Your pediatrician prescribes cephalexin, a common antibiotic. You might wonder, "Is this safe for my child?" The good news is that cephalexin is often used in children to treat various infections, including skin and respiratory infections. It's generally well-tolerated, but just like with any medication, there are a few things to keep in mind. One of the main considerations with pediatric patients is dosage. Children aren't just tiny adults; their bodies process medications differently. Doctors usually calculate the right dose based on the child's weight, ensuring they receive the proper amount without any risks. As a parent, it's vital to follow the prescribed dosage carefully and watch for any unusual reactions, like a rash or upset stomach.

You might also have heard that some antibiotics can disrupt the natural balance of bacteria in a child's gut. This is true for cephalexin as well. To help maintain a healthy gut, consider introducing some probiotics into their diet—like yogurt or supplements—after finishing the course of antibiotics. These can help restore the good bacteria that may have been affected.

Now, let's shift our focus to another group: the elderly. Imagine an older relative who has been prescribed cephalexin for a urinary tract infection. Many people worry about how medications might interact with their existing health conditions or other prescriptions they're taking. As we age, our bodies metabolize drugs differently, which can sometimes increase the risk of side effects.

For elderly patients, doctors usually start with a lower dose and monitor for any adverse effects. This cautious approach helps ensure that the benefits of the medication outweigh any potential risks. Open communication is vital here—if your elderly loved one experiences dizziness or confusion, it's crucial to contact their healthcare provider immediately.

Pregnant and breastfeeding women also fall into a unique category when it comes to medications. You might wonder if it's safe to take cephalexin during pregnancy. Generally, cephalexin is considered a safer choice for treating bacterial infections in pregnant women compared to some other antibiotics. However, it's always best to discuss any medications with a healthcare provider who can assess individual circumstances.

If a pregnant woman is prescribed cephalexin, she should also be aware of any potential side effects. While most women tolerate it well, some might experience gastrointestinal discomfort. This is a good time to remind yourself of the importance of hydration and balanced nutrition, as these can help mitigate some of those side effects. In all these scenarios, one theme stands out: the importance of vigilance and communication with healthcare providers. If you or a loved one falls into one of these special populations, it's essential to have an open dialogue with your doctor about concerns, potential side effects, and the best course of action.

Ultimately, cephalexin can be a valuable tool for treating infections in various populations when used correctly. Understanding how it affects different groups helps ensure that everyone receives safe and effective care. Remember, whether it's for your child, an elderly family member, or during pregnancy, knowledge is power. By being informed and proactive, you can navigate the world of antibiotics with confidence and care.

12.1 Use in Children

When it comes to treating infections in children, cephalexin can be a valuable tool in a parent's medicine cabinet. You might have heard stories from other parents about their kids battling everything from ear infections to skin rashes. So, let's dive into how cephalexin is used in children, what parents should know, and how to ensure the little ones stay safe and healthy. Imagine this scenario: your child has been complaining about ear pain and tugging at their ear. After a visit to the pediatrician, you learn that your child has an ear infection, a common issue for many kids. The doctor prescribes cephalexin, an antibiotic known for its effectiveness in treating various bacterial infections. You might be feeling a mix of relief and concern. Will this medication help? Is it safe?

Cephalexin is often used to treat ear infections, respiratory infections, and skin infections in children. One reason doctors choose cephalexin is that it's generally well-tolerated. Many kids take it without any significant issues. However, just like with any medication, there are a few things to keep in mind.

Dosing is a crucial part of using cephalexin in children. Unlike adults, children's bodies are still developing, so their weight plays a vital role in determining how much medication they should receive. Doctors usually prescribe cephalexin based on the child's weight to ensure they get the right amount.

For parents, this means keeping an eye on your child's growth and sharing that information with the doctor during visits. You might be thinking about the potential side effects. Many parents worry about how their kids will react to new medications. While cephalexin is typically safe, some children might experience side effects like stomach upset or diarrhea. It's helpful to keep track of how your child feels while they're on medication. If you notice any concerning symptoms, don't hesitate to call your doctor.

Speaking of side effects, it's essential to remember that antibiotics can disrupt the balance of good bacteria in the gut. This might lead to a bit of digestive trouble. To support your child's gut health, you can introduce probiotics into their diet. Foods like yogurt can help replenish those friendly bacteria, making the treatment process smoother.

You might also wonder about the duration of treatment. Typically, a course of cephalexin lasts about 7 to 14 days, depending on the infection. It's essential to complete the full course, even if your child starts feeling better before finishing the medication. Stopping early might leave some bacteria behind, potentially leading to a resurgence of the infection. Many parents find it helpful to create a routine around medication time. This could be as simple as giving the medicine right after a meal or incorporating it into a bedtime routine. Making it a regular part of their day can help ensure your child takes their medication consistently.

Lastly, it's crucial to have open conversations with your child about their treatment. Depending on their age, explaining what the medicine is for can help them understand why it's important. You could say something like, "This medicine will help make your ear feel better so you can get back to playing with your friends." Framing it positively can make a big difference in how they feel about taking their medicine.

Using cephalexin in children can be effective in treating bacterial infections when done thoughtfully. By understanding how to administer the medication properly, watching for side effects, and fostering open communication, parents can help ensure their kids get the best care possible. Remember, if you ever have questions or concerns, your pediatrician is a valuable resource, ready to help you navigate this journey.

12.2 Use During Pregnancy and Breastfeeding

When it comes to taking medications during pregnancy and breastfeeding, the stakes can feel incredibly high. If you're expecting a baby or nursing, you might find yourself in situations where a doctor prescribes a medication like cephalexin. So, what does that mean for you and your little one? Let's unpack this topic together.

Imagine you're in your third trimester, and you start to feel a familiar pain—maybe it's a toothache or an unexpected infection. You might be concerned about how taking medication could affect your baby. This is a common worry, and it's completely understandable. The good news is that cephalexin is generally considered safe for use during pregnancy. It belongs to a class of antibiotics known as cephalosporins, which have been used for many years.

Many women are relieved to learn that cephalexin has a good safety profile. Studies have shown that it doesn't pose significant risks to the developing baby. However, every pregnancy is unique, and it's essential to have a chat with your healthcare provider. They'll take into account your specific situation and help weigh the benefits of treatment against any potential risks.

Now, let's talk about breastfeeding. You might wonder if cephalexin passes into breast milk and whether it's safe for your nursing baby. While some medications do transfer into breast milk, cephalexin is generally considered safe for breastfeeding mothers. The amount that actually makes it into your milk is typically very low and unlikely to harm your baby. Still, it's a good practice to monitor your baby for any unusual signs or reactions, just to be on the safe side.

You may also be curious about how to manage infections while balancing the needs of a newborn. Picture this: you're recovering from a surgical procedure after childbirth and are prescribed cephalexin to prevent infection. Between diaper changes and late-night feedings, you're already juggling a lot. Making sure you remember to take your medication can feel daunting. Many mothers find it helpful to set a timer or use a medication app to keep track of their doses. Establishing a routine can make this part of your day feel more manageable.

Another concern many new moms have is how medication might affect their milk supply. While there's limited evidence suggesting that cephalexin impacts breastfeeding, staying hydrated and eating well is key to maintaining a healthy milk supply. It's also important to listen to your body. If you notice any changes in your breastfeeding routine, don't hesitate to reach out to a lactation consultant or your healthcare provider for guidance.

As with any medication, there might be side effects to consider. Some women report mild digestive issues while taking cephalexin, such as nausea or diarrhea. If you're experiencing these side effects, try to stay hydrated and maintain a balanced diet. Many mothers have found that eating smaller, more frequent meals helps alleviate some discomfort.

Finally, it's essential to communicate openly with your healthcare team. You might feel a bit overwhelmed by the decisions you have to make, but remember that your doctor and pharmacist are there to help. They can answer your questions, provide support, and help you navigate your treatment options safely. While taking cephalexin during pregnancy and breastfeeding can be safe, it's crucial to approach it with care and communication. Understanding the facts and having open conversations with your healthcare provider can help you make informed decisions for both you and your baby. With the right support, you can manage your health while enjoying this special time in your life.

12.3 Use in Elderly Patients

When it comes to healthcare, older adults often have unique needs and concerns, especially regarding medication like cephalexin. You might be wondering why that is. After all, many people take antibiotics without a second thought. But as we age, our bodies change in ways that can affect how we process medications. Picture this: an elderly gentleman named Mr. Thompson visits his doctor after experiencing some symptoms that might suggest a bacterial infection. Perhaps it's a persistent cough or a urinary tract infection, common issues among older adults. His doctor prescribes cephalexin, a reliable antibiotic. But you might ask, how does age influence the way Mr. Thompson's body reacts to this medication?

As we age, our liver and kidneys may not work as efficiently as they once did. These organs play a crucial role in breaking down and eliminating medications from our bodies. For Mr. Thompson, this could mean that cephalexin stays in his system longer than it would in a younger patient, potentially increasing the risk of side effects. This is why healthcare providers often start elderly patients on lower doses and closely monitor them for any reactions.

Many people worry about side effects when starting a new medication. Mr. Thompson is no exception. He's heard stories from friends about how antibiotics can cause upset stomachs or lead to yeast infections. While cephalexin is generally well-tolerated, it's important for him to be aware of these potential side effects. His doctor may suggest taking the antibiotic with food to help reduce stomach irritation, which can make a big difference in how he feels.

You might wonder how elderly patients like Mr. Thompson can manage their medications alongside other health conditions. It's common for older adults to take multiple medications for various issues like high blood pressure, diabetes, or arthritis. This is known as polypharmacy. For Mr. Thompson, keeping track of when to take each medication can feel overwhelming. That's why creating a medication schedule or using a pill organizer can be incredibly helpful. Many elderly patients find that using a simple chart or app can alleviate some of the stress of managing their medications.

Family members and caregivers play a crucial role in this process, too. For instance, Mr. Thompson's daughter might help him organize his medications and remind him when it's time to take them. Having someone to lean on can make a world of difference, especially when side effects or confusion about dosing occur.

It's also important to consider any underlying health conditions. For instance, if Mr. Thompson has diabetes, his blood sugar levels might need closer monitoring during his antibiotic treatment. In such cases, communication between healthcare providers and the patient's family can ensure that everyone is on the same page.

Another aspect to think about is how antibiotics can affect gut health. Older adults often have more sensitive digestive systems, and antibiotics can disrupt the natural balance of good bacteria in the gut. Mr. Thompson might be advised to take probiotics during and after his course of cephalexin to help restore that balance and minimize the risk of gastrointestinal upset. You might also wonder about the importance of follow-up care. After finishing his course of cephalexin, Mr. Thompson should check back in with his doctor. It's crucial to ensure that the infection has cleared up and that there are no lingering side effects. This follow-up is especially important for older patients, as their bodies may take longer to heal.

The use of cephalexin in elderly patients requires special consideration. Understanding how aging affects medication metabolism, managing potential side effects, and keeping track of other health conditions are all important factors. With the right support and a proactive approach, elderly patients like Mr. Thompson can effectively navigate their antibiotic treatment and maintain their health. By staying informed and engaged, patients and their families can work together to ensure the best possible outcomes.

CHAPTER 13

Future of Antibiotic Treatments

When you think about antibiotics, you might picture that familiar brown bottle in your medicine cabinet, filled with tiny pills that have been a staple in treating infections for decades. But as we look to the future of antibiotic treatments, it's essential to recognize that this field is evolving rapidly, facing challenges and offering exciting new possibilities.

Imagine for a moment that you're a parent with a child who has just come down with an ear infection. In the past, a quick visit to the doctor would likely end with a prescription for amoxicillin. But today, you might find yourself wondering about the future of such treatments. How will antibiotics change to keep pace with the growing problem of antibiotic resistance? One of the biggest concerns today is that many bacteria are becoming resistant to the antibiotics we currently have. This means that those once-reliable medications may not work as effectively as they used to. You might have heard stories of patients who faced severe infections due to antibiotic-resistant bacteria. These stories highlight the urgent need for new approaches and innovations in the world of antibiotics.

So, what does the future hold? Researchers are hard at work exploring various strategies to combat these resistant strains. One exciting area of development is the use of bacteriophages. You might be wondering what that means. Simply put, bacteriophages are viruses that specifically target bacteria. Think of them as tiny hunters that seek out and destroy their bacterial prey. In some cases, they can be more effective than traditional antibiotics. Imagine a treatment that tailors itself to attack specific strains of bacteria, potentially reducing the risk of resistance!

Another promising avenue is the development of new classes of antibiotics. Scientists are diving deep into the world of nature, looking for compounds in plants, fungi, and even soil that might lead to the discovery of new antibiotics. You might remember hearing about penicillin, which was discovered by accident when Alexander Fleming noticed that mold had killed bacteria in his lab. That spirit of exploration is alive today, with researchers seeking the next groundbreaking discovery in unlikely places.

You may also have heard of "combination therapies." This is when two or more antibiotics are used together to treat an infection. The idea is that by combining different mechanisms of action, we can overcome resistance. For instance, if one antibiotic isn't working, the other might be effective, or they could work together to enhance each other's effects. It's a bit like teaming up with a buddy in a game to tackle a tough level together.

You might be surprised to learn that personalized medicine is making its way into antibiotic treatments too. The concept involves tailoring medical treatment to the individual characteristics of each patient. In the future, doctors could analyze the specific bacteria causing an infection and prescribe an antibiotic that is most effective for that strain, much like how a tailor adjusts a suit to fit just right. This approach could significantly improve treatment outcomes and reduce the misuse of antibiotics.

As we explore the future, it's important to remember that education plays a crucial role in combating antibiotic resistance. You might wonder how you can help. One of the most powerful tools we have is simply being informed. Understanding when antibiotics are necessary—and when they aren't—can make a significant difference. For instance, many viral infections, like the common cold or the flu, don't respond to antibiotics. Knowing this can help you avoid unnecessary use and protect the effectiveness of these critical medications.

In the years to come, we might also see advancements in rapid diagnostic testing. Imagine walking into a doctor's office and getting results in minutes instead of days. Quick tests could help doctors determine whether an infection is bacterial or viral, allowing them to prescribe antibiotics only when necessary. This kind of innovation could be a game changer in the fight against antibiotic resistance.

The future of antibiotic treatments holds tremendous potential, filled with innovative strategies and a commitment to finding solutions. From bacteriophages to personalized medicine, these advancements could reshape how we approach infections. As you think about the next time you or your loved ones might need antibiotics, remember that the landscape is changing. By staying informed and understanding how to use antibiotics wisely, you can be a part of this critical conversation. The journey is ongoing, and the future looks promising.

13.1 Innovations in Bacterial Infection Management

When you think about how we've tackled bacterial infections over the years, it's like watching a captivating story unfold. Imagine your great-grandparents living in a world without antibiotics. A simple cut or a mild infection could lead to serious consequences. Thankfully, the invention of antibiotics transformed medicine, turning potential tragedies into manageable health issues. But as we've learned more about bacteria, we've also encountered challenges—especially with antibiotic resistance. So, what innovations are on the horizon for managing bacterial infections?

Let's take a closer look at some of the exciting developments shaping the future of bacterial infection management. You might wonder how these innovations are changing the game for everyday people, like your child dealing with an ear infection or your grandmother who frequently faces urinary tract infections (UTIs).

One area that's getting a lot of attention is **bacteriophage therapy**. Picture this: bacteriophages are tiny viruses that specifically attack bacteria, almost like a secret weapon in your medicine cabinet. Imagine if your body had a superhero that only targeted the bad guys—this is what bacteriophages do! They hunt down and destroy specific bacteria, making them a promising alternative for infections resistant to traditional antibiotics. In fact, some researchers are already using phages in clinical settings, and people are seeing positive results.

Let's say your child is prescribed antibiotics for that ear infection, but the bacteria are resistant. Instead of relying solely on antibiotics, doctors could explore using bacteriophages tailored to target that specific strain. It's like having a specialized tool for a unique problem. And as we continue to learn about these phages, the hope is that they could become a common part of infection management.

Another promising innovation comes from **combination therapies**. You might have heard of this concept before, but it's gaining traction in the fight against stubborn infections. Imagine you're making a delicious dish, and the recipe calls for more than one ingredient to achieve the best flavor. In the same way, combining different antibiotics can enhance effectiveness, especially against resistant bacteria.

For example, if your grandmother has a recurring UTI, a doctor might prescribe a combination of antibiotics to ensure a more robust attack on the bacteria causing her discomfort. This tailored approach not only targets the infection more effectively but also reduces the likelihood of bacteria becoming resistant in the first place.

You may also be interested in the advancements in **rapid diagnostic testing**. Remember those times when you had to wait for what felt like an eternity to find out what was making you sick? Well, future testing could change that. With rapid diagnostic tools, healthcare providers could identify the exact bacteria causing an infection in just minutes rather than days.

Imagine you're at the doctor's office with a suspected bacterial infection. Instead of going home with a broad-spectrum antibiotic that might not be effective, the doctor can quickly test your sample and determine the precise bacteria at play. This means you get the right treatment faster, which can lead to quicker recovery times and less chance for resistance to develop.

There's also a growing interest in **vaccines** for bacterial infections. You might already be familiar with vaccines that prevent illnesses like flu or measles, but researchers are now focusing on developing vaccines against specific bacterial infections, like pneumonia or strep throat. This is like putting on a shield to protect yourself before encountering potential threats.

For instance, if a new vaccine for strep throat becomes available, it could reduce the number of infections and, in turn, lessen the need for antibiotics. Imagine a world where kids can play without the constant worry of infections. That's a future worth striving for!

Additionally, the field of **personalized medicine** is paving the way for more effective treatment plans. You might be familiar with the concept of tailoring your diet or exercise routine to your specific needs, but the same principle applies to medicine. With advancements in genetic testing, doctors can analyze how a patient's unique biology interacts with certain medications.

This means that when you or a loved one receives a diagnosis, the treatment plan can be customized to fit your unique situation. So, if your child has an unusual reaction to a particular antibiotic, doctors could use genetic insights to select a more effective option.

As we move forward, it's clear that innovation in bacterial infection management is not just about new medications but also about using technology and knowledge to enhance patient care. From bacteriophages and combination therapies to rapid testing and personalized medicine, the future holds great promise.

Many people worry about antibiotic resistance and what it means for our health, but these innovations are part of the solution. As we learn more and adapt our approaches, we're heading toward a world where bacterial infections can be managed more effectively, keeping our families safe and healthy. So, the next time you find yourself in a doctor's office, remember that the story of antibiotics is still being written, and the future looks bright.

13.2 Trends in Antibiotic Prescribing Practices

When it comes to antibiotics, you might wonder how doctors decide what to prescribe. With so many different medications out there, trends in prescribing practices are evolving to ensure that patients receive the best care while combating the growing problem of antibiotic resistance. So, let's dive into some of these trends and how they might affect you or your loved ones.

One significant shift we're seeing is the move toward **more careful prescribing**. Many healthcare providers are becoming more aware of the risks associated with overprescribing antibiotics. Imagine a family at home dealing with a child's persistent cough. Parents might rush to the doctor, hoping for a quick fix, and antibiotics can sometimes seem like the easy answer. But in many cases, coughs are caused by viruses, not bacteria.

In the past, a doctor might have prescribed antibiotics without much thought, but now, many are taking the time to explain to parents that antibiotics won't help a viral infection. Instead, they might recommend other treatments—like rest, fluids, and a humidifier. This change isn't just about saving money; it's about preserving the effectiveness of antibiotics for when they are genuinely needed.

Another trend is **evidence-based prescribing**. You might have heard this term before, but what does it mean in practical terms? It's about using the latest research and clinical guidelines to determine the best treatment options. Imagine your grandmother visits the doctor with a UTI. In the past, doctors might have prescribed the same antibiotic every time without considering the most recent guidelines. Now, with better access to data and research, physicians are more likely to prescribe medications based on current evidence about which antibiotics are most effective for specific infections. This is particularly crucial in managing antibiotic resistance. By tailoring prescriptions to individual cases and relying on up-to-date research, doctors can help prevent bacteria from becoming resistant to commonly used treatments.

You might also notice the rise of **rapid diagnostic tests** in your local healthcare settings. These tests can quickly determine what type of bacteria is causing an infection, allowing doctors to prescribe antibiotics that are most likely to work. Picture this scenario: you or your child goes to the doctor with an infection. Instead of guessing which antibiotic might work best, the doctor can run a quick test and identify the culprit in just a few hours.

This means that when you get a prescription, it's much more likely to be the right one. It's like having a map that leads directly to the solution instead of wandering around hoping to find your way.

In addition to these advancements, there's a growing emphasis on **patient education**. Many people worry about the side effects of antibiotics or how to take them properly. Doctors are now spending more time discussing the importance of completing a prescribed course, even if you start to feel better. You might have heard someone say, "I felt fine after a few days, so I stopped taking my antibiotics."

While that might seem reasonable, it can actually lead to bacteria surviving and potentially becoming resistant. Doctors are now explaining this to patients, emphasizing that finishing the full course is crucial for both individual health and the broader fight against resistance.

Let's not forget the increasing focus on **antibiotic stewardship programs** in healthcare settings. These programs aim to ensure that antibiotics are prescribed only when necessary and that the right antibiotics are used for the right infections. In hospitals, this might mean a team of healthcare providers reviews antibiotic prescriptions regularly, ensuring that patients receive the best possible treatment. Think of it like having a safety net; if a doctor prescribes an antibiotic, another team member checks to see if it's appropriate. This collaboration helps reduce unnecessary prescriptions and keeps patients safer.

Finally, there's a noticeable trend toward **alternative therapies** for infections. While antibiotics are essential, some healthcare providers are exploring complementary treatments. You might be curious about options like probiotics, which can help restore healthy gut bacteria after antibiotic treatment. These alternatives are becoming more common as research continues to unveil their benefits.

As we look to the future, it's evident that antibiotic prescribing practices are evolving to meet new challenges. The focus is shifting toward responsible prescribing, better diagnostics, and education, all aimed at preserving the effectiveness of antibiotics. So, the next time you or a loved one is dealing with an infection, know that healthcare providers are working diligently to ensure that the best possible treatment is being offered, keeping you safe while fighting bacteria effectively. The journey of antibiotics continues, and with these trends, there's hope for a healthier tomorrow.

Conclusion

As we wrap up our exploration of antibiotics, it's essential to reflect on what we've learned about these powerful medications and their role in our health. You might be thinking about the last time you or a loved one needed antibiotics. Perhaps it was for a stubborn ear infection in your child or a urinary tract infection for an elderly relative. These experiences highlight how antibiotics can be lifesavers, turning what could be a severe health issue into a manageable one.

However, it's crucial to remember that with great power comes great responsibility. While antibiotics like cephalexin can be incredibly effective, we must use them wisely. The rise of antibiotic resistance is a concern we all share, and understanding when and how to use these medications is vital for our collective health.

Moving forward, it's clear that innovation in antibiotic treatments and thoughtful prescribing practices will shape the future of healthcare. By embracing evidence-based approaches, rapid diagnostic testing, and patient education, we can ensure that antibiotics remain effective tools in our medical arsenal.

So, whether you're a parent, a caregiver, or simply someone interested in health, staying informed about antibiotics is essential. As we continue to navigate the complexities of bacterial infections, let's prioritize informed choices and support practices that promote the responsible use of these medications. Together, we can help safeguard the future of antibiotic treatments for generations to come.

Key Takeaways for Safe Use

When it comes to using antibiotics safely, a few key takeaways can help guide your decisions and ensure you're getting the most from these vital medications. Whether you're a parent worried about your child's health or someone managing your own condition, understanding how to use antibiotics responsibly is essential.

First and foremost, only use antibiotics when prescribed by a healthcare professional. You might wonder why this is important, especially if you feel tempted to self-diagnose and treat minor infections at home. The reality is that antibiotics are specifically designed to tackle bacterial infections, not viral ones like colds or the flu. Using them inappropriately can lead to resistance, meaning that the next time you really need antibiotics, they might not work as effectively.

If you do receive a prescription, make sure to follow the dosage instructions carefully. Completing the full course of antibiotics, even if you start to feel better before it's finished, is crucial. Stopping early can allow some bacteria to survive, which can lead to a resurgence of the infection and contribute to antibiotic resistance. Picture this: it's like not finishing a puzzle—some pieces may be missing, and the whole picture won't come together.

For families, it's important to keep an eye on potential side effects. You may have experienced or heard stories about mild side effects like stomach upset or rashes, which are relatively common. However, if you notice severe reactions, such as difficulty breathing or swelling, don't hesitate to seek medical attention right away. This vigilance can help ensure everyone stays safe.

Also, consider the broader impact of antibiotic use. The choices you make can affect not just your health but also the health of your community. Sharing information with friends and family about the responsible use of antibiotics can help create a ripple effect, leading to better health outcomes for everyone.

Lastly, stay informed. Regular check-ins with your healthcare provider about antibiotic use can provide clarity on when they're truly necessary. This ongoing dialogue can help you feel empowered and knowledgeable, making you an advocate for your own health and the health of those around you.

In summary, using antibiotics safely involves understanding their purpose, following medical advice, being aware of side effects, and keeping the bigger picture in mind. By taking these steps, you can play a vital role in preserving the effectiveness of antibiotics for yourself and future generations.

Final Words of Encouragement

As we wrap up our journey through the world of antibiotics, I want to leave you with some encouraging words. Navigating health issues can sometimes feel overwhelming, especially when you're trying to figure out the best course of action for yourself or a loved one. Remember, you're not alone in this.

Many people find themselves in similar situations—like that time your child came home from school with a nasty ear infection. You might recall the worried look on their face, and the relief that washed over you when the doctor prescribed amoxicillin. It's a common story, and it highlights how important it is to understand the medications we use.

You might be wondering how to make the most out of your healthcare experiences. Start by asking questions. Don't hesitate to seek clarity from your healthcare provider. They want to help you feel informed and confident about your treatment plan.

It's perfectly okay to express your concerns and ensure you understand the why behind your prescription. Let's not forget that the path to better health often involves more than just medication. Healthy lifestyle choices—like eating a balanced diet, staying active, and getting enough rest—play a huge role in how your body fights off infections. You can think of your body as a team, where each player—nutrition, exercise, and rest—works together to keep you strong.

And as you think about your role in this, consider the impact of responsible antibiotic use. When you choose to use antibiotics wisely, you're contributing to a healthier future for everyone. Imagine a world where antibiotics remain effective, protecting not just you and your family but also the broader community. That's a powerful goal.

So, as you move forward, stay curious and proactive about your health. Equip yourself with knowledge, lean on your support system, and remember that every small step counts. You've got the tools you need to make informed choices, and that's something to feel empowered about. Keep advocating for yourself and your loved ones, and trust that with care and attention, you can navigate the complexities of health with confidence.

FAQs and Common Concerns (Bonus)

When it comes to taking antibiotics, many people have questions and concerns. You might be wondering if you're alone in feeling a little anxious about it all. Let's dive into some frequently asked questions to clear up common worries and make this topic a bit easier to digest. You might have heard that antibiotics can lead to side effects. This is true, but they vary from person to person. Some folks might experience mild stomach upset, while others may feel a bit dizzy or even break out in a rash. It's always a good idea to communicate with your doctor if you notice anything unusual. They can help you weigh the benefits of the medication against any potential side effects.

Another common concern is whether antibiotics will work for every infection. This is where understanding bacteria versus viruses comes in handy. For instance, you wouldn't take amoxicillin for the flu, because that's caused by a virus, not bacteria. Many people worry about taking antibiotics unnecessarily, and they have a right to—overuse can lead to antibiotic resistance, which is a growing problem. It's like if everyone kept pushing the same button, eventually, it just wouldn't work anymore. You might also wonder if it's safe to use antibiotics during pregnancy or while breastfeeding. Many doctors consider amoxicillin a safer option, but it's essential to have a chat with your healthcare provider. They can give you tailored advice based on your specific situation, helping you feel more at ease.

A scenario many parents can relate to is when their child gets a common illness, like an ear infection. You might be anxious to get the right treatment, but remember, not all ear infections require antibiotics. Sometimes, doctors might suggest a wait-and-see approach. This can be tough, especially when your little one is uncomfortable, but it's often the best choice. You might also worry about what happens if you miss a dose of your antibiotic. If you forget to take it, don't panic. Just take it as soon as you remember, unless it's close to the time for your next dose. In that case, skip the missed one and carry on with your schedule. It's a good idea to set reminders or use a pill organizer to help keep you on track. Lastly, let's touch on the importance of completing your prescribed course of antibiotics. Many people think, "I feel better, so I can stop taking these." But that's a bit like leaving a job half-finished. Stopping early can allow bacteria to survive and potentially become resistant to the medication. This is why your doctor emphasizes finishing the entire course.

So, as you navigate your antibiotic journey, remember you're not alone. It's natural to have questions and concerns. Trust in your healthcare team, stay informed, and don't hesitate to ask for help when you need it. By staying engaged and proactive, you can make informed decisions about your health and feel more confident along the way.

Can Cephalexin Be Used for Viral Infections?

You might be curious if cephalexin, an antibiotic commonly used to treat bacterial infections, can also be used for viral infections. It's a question that many people have, especially when they're feeling under the weather and just want to feel better quickly.

First, let's clear up some terminology. Cephalexin belongs to a class of antibiotics called cephalosporins, and it works by fighting bacteria. When you have a bacterial infection—like a strep throat or a skin infection—cephalexin can be a helpful tool to help your body fight off those pesky bacteria. However, it's important to know that antibiotics like cephalexin do not work against viruses. So, if you catch a cold or the flu, which are viral infections, taking cephalexin won't do you any good. It's a bit like trying to fix a flat tire with a hammer; it just won't work.

You might wonder why this distinction is important. Many people rush to the doctor when they feel sick, hoping for a quick fix. Imagine a parent taking their child to the doctor for a runny nose and cough. The doctor examines the child and determines it's a viral infection. If the parent requests antibiotics, it's crucial for the doctor to explain why they won't help. This is not just about following protocol; it's about preventing antibiotic resistance, a growing concern in the medical community. When antibiotics are overprescribed or used inappropriately, they can become less effective over time.

You might have heard stories about someone who took antibiotics for a viral infection and didn't feel better. This can be frustrating and may lead to a cycle of taking more medications without understanding what's happening. For example, let's say you catch a nasty stomach virus. You might be tempted to ask for cephalexin, hoping it will ease your symptoms. But in reality, the best approach is often rest, hydration, and time. Your body is resilient, and it knows how to fight off viruses.

In some cases, people might experience a secondary bacterial infection following a viral illness. For instance, after having the flu, a person may develop a sinus infection. In such cases, a doctor might prescribe cephalexin to tackle the new bacterial infection. This is an important distinction because it highlights how antibiotics should only be used when there's a clear bacterial component.

While cephalexin is effective against bacterial infections, it's not the answer for viral infections. If you find yourself wondering about the best course of action when you're feeling ill, don't hesitate to consult your healthcare provider. They can help guide you toward the right treatment, ensuring that you stay healthy without contributing to antibiotic resistance. It's all about using the right tool for the job and trusting your body's ability to heal.

What If My Symptoms Improve Before the Course Ends?

How Long Does It Stay in the System?

You might be wondering how long cephalexin stays in your system after you finish taking it. This is an important question, especially if you're managing your health or preparing for a procedure.

Let's break it down in simple terms. Cephalexin is a type of antibiotic, and like many medications, it doesn't just disappear from your body the moment you stop taking it. Instead, it has a half-life, which is the time it takes for half of the drug to be eliminated from your system. For cephalexin, this half-life is generally around 1 to 2 hours, but several factors can influence how long it stays in your system. You might be thinking about a common scenario, like when your child has a severe ear infection. After the doctor prescribes cephalexin, you dutifully give it to them for a full week. But once the treatment ends, when can you expect the medication to be fully cleared from their system? Generally, it takes about 5 to 6 half-lives for a drug to be eliminated, so you can expect cephalexin to be out of your child's system within about 6 to 12 hours after the last dose. That's pretty quick, right?

However, individual factors come into play here. Age, kidney function, and overall health can affect how long cephalexin lingers in your system. For instance, if an elderly person or someone with kidney issues is taking cephalexin, it might take longer for their body to clear the medication. This is why healthcare providers always take a detailed medical history before prescribing medications.

You might recall hearing stories about friends who felt side effects lingered long after they finished their antibiotics. That's not uncommon! Even when the drug is out of your bloodstream, some side effects can take a little longer to subside. If someone experienced stomach upset or diarrhea during treatment, they might continue to feel that way for a bit longer, even after cephalexin has cleared their system. If you ever have concerns about how long a medication might last in your body, don't hesitate to reach out to your healthcare provider. They can give you personalized advice based on your health history and the specific medications you're taking.

While cephalexin generally leaves the body fairly quickly, individual factors can affect how long it stays in your system. It's always good to stay informed and to communicate with your healthcare provider about any questions or concerns you may have. After all, your health is a partnership, and understanding your treatment is a key part of that journey.

Resources and Further Reading

When it comes to understanding antibiotics like cephalexin or amoxicillin, you might be looking for more information to help navigate your questions. It's always good to be informed, especially when it comes to your health or the health of someone you care about. Here are some resources and further reading options that can help you dive deeper into the world of antibiotics.

First off, let's talk about the basics. The **Centers for Disease Control and Prevention (CDC)** has a fantastic website that covers everything you need to know about antibiotics, including their use, side effects, and the growing concern of antibiotic resistance. You might be surprised to learn how often antibiotics are prescribed and why it's essential to use them responsibly.

Another great resource is the **World Health Organization (WHO)**, which has numerous publications about antibiotic stewardship. They provide insight into how countries are tackling antibiotic resistance on a global scale, which might feel a bit daunting at first but is crucial information if you want to understand the bigger picture.

If you're interested in the science behind antibiotics, consider picking up a book like **"The Antibiotic Era: Reform, Resistance, and the Pursuit of the Perfect Drug"** by Elinor Clare. This book walks you through the history of antibiotics, offering personal stories and anecdotes that make the complex science more relatable. You'll find yourself immersed in the journey of how these life-saving medications were discovered and developed.

For practical, everyday advice, **MedlinePlus** offers a user-friendly resource that explains different medications, including cephalexin. They break down dosages, side effects, and potential interactions in a way that's easy to digest. You might find it helpful, especially if you're managing a child's ear infection or looking after an elderly relative.

You might also want to check out **Consumer Reports Health**, which frequently publishes articles on how to use antibiotics wisely. They emphasize the importance of discussing any concerns with your doctor, especially when it comes to side effects or if the prescribed antibiotic doesn't seem to be working.

Lastly, joining a local or online support group can be incredibly beneficial. Many communities have forums where people share their experiences with different medications. Hearing others' stories can be comforting and provide practical tips that you might not find in books or articles.

Remember, it's always good to ask questions. Whether you're reading articles, consulting your healthcare provider, or joining a community, the more informed you are, the better equipped you'll be to make decisions about your health. So, take your time exploring these resources and feel confident in your understanding of antibiotics and their role in healthcare. You're not alone on this journey!

Trusted Online Health Resources

In today's digital age, finding reliable health information online can feel like searching for a needle in a haystack. With so much information at our fingertips, it's important to know which sources you can trust, especially when it comes to understanding medications like amoxicillin or cephalexin.

You might wonder where to start. One excellent resource is the **Mayo Clinic website**. It's well-known for its clear, concise information about various health topics, including detailed descriptions of different medications. For instance, if you're trying to figure out whether to give amoxicillin to your child for an ear infection, the Mayo Clinic can guide you through the dosages, side effects, and even offer practical tips for ensuring your child feels comfortable during treatment. Another fantastic resource is **WebMD**. While it's easy to get lost in the numerous articles, their "Medication" section is particularly user-friendly. They often break down complex medical jargon into simple terms. For example, if you read about cephalexin, you'll find straightforward explanations of what it treats, how it works, and what side effects to watch for. Plus, the forums can provide a sense of community where people share their personal experiences. Hearing how others navigated similar situations can be reassuring.

If you're curious about a broader perspective on health, the **Centers for Disease Control and Prevention (CDC)** has a wealth of information, especially on public health concerns like antibiotic resistance. You might find articles detailing the importance of taking antibiotics correctly and the dangers of misuse, such as why it's critical to finish the prescribed course even if you feel better. It's a great way to understand the bigger picture of how our actions impact community health.

For a more interactive experience, consider checking out **Healthline**. Their articles often include infographics and videos that explain health topics in an engaging way. If you're wondering how to properly use antibiotics, Healthline can guide you through the process with relatable examples. Think about how you might need to explain the importance of completing a course of antibiotics to a family member who might be skeptical—these resources can give you the right words to say.

You may also want to look into **PubMed Health** for research-based articles. This site provides summaries of medical studies, making it easier for you to understand the latest findings in a way that's not overwhelming. You might come across a study that highlights the effectiveness of cephalexin for treating certain infections, giving you confidence in the treatment plan your doctor suggested.

Lastly, if you're looking for community support, don't overlook **Facebook groups** or local health forums. Many people share their experiences and offer advice based on personal journeys, whether it's managing side effects or figuring out when to seek further medical help. Connecting with others can make a huge difference when you're facing a health concern. Remember, when you're online looking for health information, it's always wise to double-check your sources. The right information can empower you to make informed decisions about your health and the health of your loved ones. So take a moment to explore these trusted resources. You'll likely find valuable insights that help clarify your questions and worries, putting you on the path to better understanding your health.

Books and Articles on Antibiotics and Infection Management

When it comes to understanding antibiotics and managing infections, having the right resources at your fingertips can make all the difference. Whether you're a healthcare professional, a concerned parent, or just someone wanting to know more about how these medications work, there are some great books and articles that can provide valuable insights.

You might be wondering where to start. A fantastic book that many people find helpful is "*Antibiotics Simplified*" by Jason C. Gallagher and Conan E.

O'Brien. It's designed for both healthcare providers and everyday readers who want to understand antibiotics better. The authors break down complex topics into bite-sized pieces, making it easier to grasp the essentials. They include relatable examples, like explaining why a child might need amoxicillin for an ear infection, which can help you visualize the scenarios.

Another excellent read is "*The Antibiotic Paradox*" by Dr. Stuart B. Levy. This book dives into the history of antibiotics and the challenges we face with antibiotic resistance today. It reads almost like a thriller, full of anecdotes and real-life stories that illustrate how antibiotics have shaped medicine. You'll learn why it's so crucial to use antibiotics responsibly, especially in light of rising resistance. Many readers find themselves reflecting on their own experiences with antibiotics after reading this book, making it a truly eye-opening journey.

For those interested in articles rather than books, consider checking out resources like the *American Academy of Pediatrics*' website. They often publish articles that tackle common infections in children and the recommended antibiotic treatments. If you have a little one dealing with a recurring cough or fever, these articles can be reassuring and informative. You might find practical tips on recognizing when an antibiotic is necessary and when it's better to let the body heal on its own.

You might also be curious about how antibiotics are evolving. The article *"The Future of Antibiotics"* published in *Nature Reviews Microbiology* provides insights into cutting-edge research on new antibiotic development. It discusses the challenges researchers face and the promising new treatments on the horizon. Even if you don't have a scientific background, the article does a great job of explaining complex topics in a way that's engaging and relatable.

If you're looking for something more community-oriented, consider exploring *Patient.info*. This site offers a wealth of articles written in straightforward language about various infections and their treatments. You might stumble upon personal stories from people who've battled infections, sharing their journeys and the role antibiotics played in their recovery. These narratives can make you feel less alone in your own health concerns. You might wonder about the importance of understanding infection management. Books like *"Managing Infectious Diseases in Child Care and Schools"* by the American Academy of Pediatrics can be incredibly useful for parents and educators alike. It covers practical strategies for preventing and managing infections in group settings, making it a great resource for anyone looking to keep children healthy in schools or daycare environments.

Finally, don't overlook the power of audiobooks and podcasts. There are plenty of podcasts focused on healthcare topics that often include episodes dedicated to antibiotics and infection management. Listening to experts discuss these subjects can make the information more digestible and even entertaining.

Incorporating these resources into your reading list can deepen your understanding of antibiotics and how they work. Whether you're looking to support a loved one with an infection or simply want to be more informed about medications, these books and articles can serve as your guide. Remember, knowledge is power, especially when it comes to making informed decisions about health. So grab a book, dive into an article, or tune into a podcast, and take that next step in your journey to understanding antibiotics and infection management.

Glossary of Terms

When diving into the world of antibiotics, you may come across some terms that feel a bit intimidating. Don't worry! I'm here to break things down into simple, relatable language so you can feel confident in your understanding. Let's explore some key terms you might encounter on your journey.

Antibiotic: This is the big one! Antibiotics are medications designed to fight bacterial infections. You might think of them as your body's sidekick in the battle against illness. For example, if your child has a painful ear infection, a doctor may prescribe amoxicillin to help clear up the infection and relieve their discomfort.

Bacteria vs. Virus: It's easy to mix these two up. Bacteria are tiny living organisms that can multiply and cause infections. Think of them as the villains that need to be defeated. On the other hand, viruses are even smaller and require a living host to survive. Common cold and flu symptoms are often caused by viruses. Antibiotics like amoxicillin won't help with viral infections, which is why it's important to know the difference.

Resistance: This term is becoming more common in discussions about antibiotics. Resistance occurs when bacteria change in response to the use of antibiotics, making the medication less effective. Imagine you're trying to break into a locked door (the bacteria), and over time, the door gets a better lock (resistance). This is why it's so crucial to use antibiotics only when necessary and as directed by a healthcare professional.

Spectrum of Activity: This phrase refers to the range of bacteria that an antibiotic can effectively treat. Some antibiotics, like amoxicillin, have a broad spectrum of activity, meaning they can target a variety of bacteria. Others are narrow-spectrum and are effective against specific types. This is like having a Swiss Army knife (broad spectrum) versus a single-purpose tool (narrow spectrum).

Side Effects: Just like any medication, antibiotics can come with side effects. These might include nausea, diarrhea, or a rash. You might be wondering why these happen. Well, antibiotics not only target harmful bacteria but can also affect the beneficial bacteria in your gut. It's like accidentally knocking over a few good apples while trying to get rid of the bad ones.

Probiotics: Speaking of good bacteria, probiotics are supplements or foods that contain beneficial bacteria. Many people choose to take probiotics after finishing a course of antibiotics to help restore balance in their gut. It's like planting new seeds in a garden after a storm.

Dosage: This term simply refers to the amount of medication you should take. Your doctor will prescribe a specific dosage based on your condition, age, and overall health. Following the prescribed dosage is crucial for effective treatment and reducing the risk of resistance.

Administration Route: This just means how the antibiotic is taken. Some are swallowed as pills, while others might be given as an injection or intravenously (directly into the bloodstream). Depending on the severity of an infection, the route can make a big difference in how quickly the medication works.

Infection: This is the result of harmful bacteria or viruses invading your body and multiplying. Symptoms can vary widely, from a simple sore throat to something more serious like pneumonia. Think of an infection as an uninvited guest who overstays their welcome, causing trouble until they're shown the door.

Culture and Sensitivity Testing: This is a lab test that helps doctors determine which bacteria are causing an infection and which antibiotics will be effective against them. It's a bit like detective work—collecting clues to figure out the best way to treat the problem.

Understanding these terms can empower you in conversations about health and treatment options. You might find yourself discussing a family member's recent infection or explaining to a friend why antibiotics won't work for their cold. By demystifying the language around antibiotics, you can feel more equipped to make informed decisions about your health and the health of your loved ones. Remember, the more you know, the better you can advocate for yourself and those you care about!

Common Medical Terms Explained

Navigating the world of medicine can sometimes feel like entering a foreign land filled with complex terminology. But don't worry! I'm here to guide you through some common medical terms, making them easy to understand and relatable.

Let's start with the term **diagnosis**. You might hear this word when a doctor examines your symptoms and determines what illness you might have. For example, if your child has been tugging at their ear and complaining of pain, the doctor may diagnose them with an ear infection. It's like solving a mystery—using clues (symptoms) to find the culprit (the illness).

Then there's a symptom, which refers to any indication that something isn't quite right in the body. Symptoms can vary widely. You might experience a fever, a headache, or even a runny nose. Think of symptoms as the body's way of sending a message, saying, "Hey, something's off here!" When you recognize these signs, you can seek help sooner rather than later.

Another term you might come across is **treatment**. This refers to the methods used to help a person recover from an illness. Treatments can range from medications, like amoxicillin for a bacterial infection, to lifestyle changes, such as diet and exercise. Imagine treatment as the action plan to get back to feeling your best, like a coach developing strategies for a winning game.

You might also hear the word **prescription** thrown around. This is a written order from a doctor that tells you what medicine to take, how much, and for how long. When your doctor prescribes amoxicillin for that ear infection, they're essentially giving you a specific game plan for how to tackle the bacteria causing the problem.

Now, let's talk about **side effects**. These are unintended reactions that can occur when taking medication. For instance, while amoxicillin is great at fighting infections, it can sometimes lead to stomach upset or a rash in some people. It's important to be aware of these side effects so you can talk to your doctor if they happen. Think of side effects like unexpected bumps in the road during a smooth drive—while you're still moving forward, it can be a bit bumpy!

Allergy is another term you might encounter, especially in relation to medications. An allergy occurs when your immune system overreacts to a substance, leading to symptoms like rashes or difficulty breathing. If someone has a known allergy to penicillin (a related antibiotic), they must avoid amoxicillin to prevent serious reactions. It's like having a particular food that just doesn't sit right with you—staying away from it is key!

You may also hear the term **antibiotic resistance**. This happens when bacteria adapt over time and become immune to the effects of antibiotics. You might wonder how this occurs. Well, imagine a superhero (the antibiotic) fighting a villain (the bacteria). If the villain learns the superhero's weaknesses, they can become harder to defeat. This is why it's crucial to take antibiotics only as prescribed and finish the entire course, even if you start feeling better.

Finally, let's discuss **follow-up appointments**. After a treatment plan is initiated, your doctor may schedule follow-up visits to see how well it's working. For example, after your child finishes their course of amoxicillin, a follow-up appointment might be scheduled to ensure the ear infection is gone. It's like checking in after a project to see if everything is on track and if any adjustments need to be made.

Understanding these common medical terms can empower you in conversations about health and treatment options. The next time you visit the doctor or hear someone talk about a health issue, you'll be able to engage more meaningfully. Just remember, the journey to better health often starts with clear communication and understanding. So, whether it's about ear infections or antibiotics, knowing the lingo makes it a lot easier to navigate the healthcare world!

www.ingramcontent.com/pod-product-compliance
Lightning Source LLC
Chambersburg PA
CBHW052148220526
45471CB00004B/1575